PET Imaging of Infection and Inflammation

Guest Editors

ABASS ALAVI, MD, PhD (Hon), DSc (Hon)
HONGMING ZHUANG, MD, PhD

PET CLINICS

www.pet.theclinics.com

Consulting Editor
ABASS ALAVI, MD, PhD (Hon), DSc (Hon)

April 2012 • Volume 7 • Number 2

SAUNDERS an imprint of ELSEVIER, Inc.

W.B. SAUNDERS COMPANY
A Division of Elsevier Inc.

1600 John F. Kennedy Boulevard ● Suite 1800 ● Philadelphia, Pennsylvania 19103-2899

http://www.theclinics.com

PET CLINICS Volume 7, Number 2
April 2012 ISSN 1556-8598, ISBN-13: 978-1-4557-3916-5

Editor: Sarah Barth
Developmental Editor: Donald Mumford

PET Clinics (ISSN 1556-8598) is published quarterly by Elsevier Inc., 360 Park Avenue South, New York, NY 10010-1710. Months of issue are January, April, July, and October. Periodicals postage paid at New York, NY, and additional mailing offices. Subscription prices per year are $215.00 (US individuals), $297.00 (US institutions), $110.00 (US students), $244.00 (Canadian individuals), $332.00 (Canadian institutions), $124.00 (Canadian students), $260.00 (foreign individuals), $332.00 (foreign institutions), and $134.00 (foreign students). To receive student and resident rate, orders must be accompanied by name of affiliated institution, date of term, and the signature of program/residency coordinator on institution letterhead. Orders will be billed at individual rate until proof of status is received. Foreign air speed delivery is included in all Clinics subscription prices. All prices are subject to change without notice. POSTMASTER: Send address changes to PET Clinics, Elsevier Health Sciences Division, Subscription Customer Service, 3251 Riverport Lane, Maryland Heights, MO 63043. **Customer Service: 1-800-654-2452 (U.S. and Canada); 314-447-8871 (outside U.S. and Canada). Fax: 314-447-8029. E-mail: journalscustomerservice-usa@elsevier.com (for print support); journalsonlinesupport-usa@elsevier.com (for online support).**

Reprints. For copies of 100 or more of articles in this publication, please contact the Commercial Reprints Department, Elsevier Inc., 360 Park Avenue South, New York, NY 10010-1710. Tel.: 212-633-3812; Fax: 212-462-1935; E-mail: reprints@elsevier.com.

Printed and bound by CPI Group (UK) Ltd, Croydon, CR0 4YY

Transferred to Digital Print 2012

Contributors

CONSULTING EDITOR

ABASS ALAVI, MD, PhD (Hon), DSc (Hon)
Professor of Radiology, Division of Nuclear
Medicine, University of Pennsylvania School
of Medicine, Philadelphia, Pennsylvania

GUEST EDITORS

ABASS ALAVI, MD, PhD (Hon), DSc (Hon)
Professor of Radiology, Division of Nuclear
Medicine, University of Pennsylvania School
of Medicine, Philadelphia, Pennsylvania

HONGMING ZHUANG, MD, PhD
Associate Professor, Division of Nuclear
Medicine, Department of Radiology, Children's
Hospital of Philadelphia; Associate Professor,
Department of Radiology, Hospital of the
University of Pennsylvania, Philadelphia,
Pennsylvania

AUTHORS

ABASS ALAVI, MD, PhD (Hon), DSc (Hon)
Professor of Radiology, Division of Nuclear
Medicine, University of Pennsylvania School
of Medicine, Philadelphia, Pennsylvania

**SANDIP BASU, MBBS (Hons), DRM,
DNB, MNAMS**
Radiation Medicine Centre, Bhabha Atomic
Research Centre, Tata Memorial Hospital
Annexe, Parel, Bombay, India

QI CAO, MD, PhD
Department of Diagnostic Radiology & Nuclear
Medicine, University of Maryland School of
Medicine, Baltimore, Maryland

WENGEN CHEN, MD, PhD
Department of Diagnostic Radiology & Nuclear
Medicine, University of Maryland School of
Medicine, Baltimore, Maryland

ION CODREANU, MD, PhD
Division of Nuclear Medicine, Department
of Radiology, The Children's Hospital of
Philadelphia, University of Pennsylvania
School of Medicine, Philadelphia,
Pennsylvania

PHYLLIS DIOGUARDI, MD, MA
Division of Nuclear Medicine, Department
of Radiology, Hospital of the University of
Pennsylvania, Philadelphia, Pennsylvania

MOHAN DOSS, PhD, MCCPM
Nuclear Medicine/PET Service, Department
of Diagnostic Imaging, Fox Chase Cancer
Center, Philadelphia, Pennsylvania

SANTOSH R. GADDAM, MD
Division of Nuclear Medicine, Department
of Radiology, Hospital of the University of
Pennsylvania, Philadelphia, Pennsylvania

ROLAND HUSTINX, MD, PhD
Professor of Nuclear Medicine, Division
of Nuclear Medicine, University Hospital
of Liège, University of Liège, Liège,
Belgium

SELLAM KARUNANITHI, MD
Department of Nuclear Medicine,
All India Institute of Medical Sciences,
New Delhi, India

RAKESH KUMAR, MD, PhD
Additional Professor, Department of Nuclear Medicine, All India Institute of Medical Sciences, New Delhi, India

YUEJIAN LIU, MD
Department of Hematology, Nanfang Hospital, Southern Medical University, Guangzhou, Guangdong Province, China

MOLLY PARSONS, BA
Department of Radiology, School of Medicine, University of Pennsylvania, Philadelphia, Pennsylvania

BABAK SABOURY, MD, MPH
Department of Radiology, School of Medicine, University of Pennsylvania, Philadelphia, Pennsylvania

SABAH SERVAES, MD
Department of Radiology, The Children's Hospital of Philadelphia, University of Pennsylvania School of Medicine, Philadelphia, Pennsylvania

DREW A. TORIGIAN, MD, MA
Department of Radiology, Hospital of the University of Pennsylvania, Philadelphia, Pennsylvania

BING XU, MD, PhD
Department of Hematology, Nanfang Hospital, Southern Medical University, Guangzhou, Guangdong Province, China

JIGANG YANG, MD, PhD
Department of Nuclear Medicine, Beijing Friendship Hospital of Capital Medical University, Beijing, China; Department of Radiology, The Children's Hospital of Philadelphia, University of Pennsylvania School of Medicine, Philadelphia, Pennsylvania

JIAN Q. YU, MD, FRCPC
Chief, Nuclear Medicine/PET Service, Associate Professor, Department of Diagnostic Imaging, Fox Chase Cancer Center, Philadelphia, Pennsylvania

HONGMING ZHUANG, MD, PhD
Associate Professor, Division of Nuclear Medicine, Department of Radiology, Children's Hospital of Philadelphia; Associate Professor, Department of Radiology, Hospital of the University of Pennsylvania, Philadelphia, Pennsylvania

POUYA ZIAI, MD
Department of Radiology, School of Medicine, University of Pennsylvania, Philadelphia, Pennsylvania

Contents

A number of diagnostic tests is often necessary to differentiate aseptic loosening from periprosthetic infection in most clinical settings. The accuracy of [18F]Fluoro-deoxyglucose examined with positron emission tomography imaging (FDG PET) in diagnosing periprosthetic infection has been determined by a number of investigations. In general, Images are considered positive for infection if they demonstrate increased FDG activity at the bone-prosthesis interface of the prostheses. Based on the large number of reports in the literature the sensitivity and specificity for FDG PET are about 85–90%. The overall accuracy of this non-invasive imaging modality is superior to the other existing imaging techniques. Therefore, FDG PET appears a very promising and accurate diagnosing tool for distinguishing septic from aseptic painful hip prostheses.

This article reviews the published data on the utilization of [18F]Fluorodeoxyglucose (FDG) positron emission tomography (PET) and PET/CT imaging in patients with complicated diabetic foot. Three areas have been identified where FDG-PET/CT can have an important role in the clinical decision making process of this disease and could be helpful to the podiatricians if found accurate: (a) Diagnosis of deep soft tissue infection and osteomyelitis (OM), (b) differentiating Charcot arthropathy from OM and (c) evaluating the ischemia/atherogenesis component in a particular case. The main focus of the research initiatives involving PET in the setting of diabetic foot syndrome has been its possible role in the reliable diagnosis or exclusion of OM. The literature on the efficacy of FDG PET in reliably diagnosing or excluding OM in diabetic foot is divided with two groups of results; four studies emphasizing the potential usefulness and two depicting relatively low sensitivity of this modality. The combined PET/CT fusion approach appears better than FDG PET imaging alone owing to superior anatomical localization and thereby better differentiation of soft tissue infection and bone. With the establishment of clinically functioning PET/MRI units, it is essential to conduct further research studies designed to investigate the ability of this modality as the most optimal *one-stop shop* diagnostic imaging technique for the management of patients with diabetic foot. A relatively less explored area is the role of FDG PET in assessing atherosclerosis in the large vessels of the lower limb that could help in studying the ischemia component and its contribution in the development of diabetic foot. Further research is required in this direction.

This article discusses the role of [18F]Fluorodeoxyglucose (FDG) PET and PET/ computed tomography in diagnosis and therapeutic response assessment for the management of patients with osteomyelitis, to increase awareness of imaging pit-falls and to improve understanding of specific technical and diagnostic challenges in patients with posttraumatic chronic osteomyelitis, spinal infections, prosthetic joint infections, and diabetic foot infections. This article focuses on the usefulness of modern imaging modalities in the setting of suspected infection or inflammation and on the role of FDG-PET in the management of patients with suspected or con-firmed infection in the bones.

Despite advances in medicine in the past decades, fever of unknown origin (FUO) remains a challenging and common clinical problem. There are many different etiol-ogies for FUO. Positron emission tomography/computed tomography (PET/CT) is a powerful technique that has been proven to be useful in elucidating processes that may present as FUO. This article reviews the utility of PET/CT imaging in the evaluation of FUO, with attention to the pediatric population.

Sarcoidosis as a distinct disease entity was diagnosed more than 100 years ago. The signs and symptoms of the disease are nonspecific, posing a challenge for early and accurate diagnosis. IgG4 disease or syndrome has various clinical manifesta-tions, such as sclerosing pancreatitis, sclerosing cholangitis, prostatitis, tubuloin-terstitial nephritis, interstitial pneumonia, and enlargement of salivary glands. This article discusses the role of the different diagnostic imaging modalities in sarcoidosis and IgG4 disease, including radiographs, computed tomography, magnetic reso-nance imaging, and conventional nuclear medicine, with a special emphasis on pos-itron emission tomography as a superior modality for assessing these inflammatory diseases.

[18F]Fluorodeoxyglucose (FDG)-PET/computed tomography has become an estab-lished modality. High-resolution PET images are superior to those provided by most single-photon–emitting tracers. Apart from its value for diagnosing and restaging malignancies, PET is increasingly used to detect associated infectious and inflam-matory conditions in oncology patients. Infectious and inflammatory conditions commonly have a lower degree of FDG uptake compared with malignant lesions. In recent years the usefulness of FDG PET in differentiating coexisting infections in patients with malignancy has received only limited attention in the literature and requires further development.

Inflammatory bowel diseases (IBD) are chronic immune mediated inflammatory dis-eases that affect the gastrointestinal tract. Two distinct entities are recognized: Crohn disease (CD) and ulcerative colitis (UC). Both entities are chronic relapsing diseases. Therapeutic algorithms have been deeply changed in recent years, thanks to the advent of biologic drugs. Nevertheless, several major questions persist regarding the clinical management of these diseases. FDG PET/CT is highly sensitive for identifying severe to moderate inflammatory involvement of the digestive tract. Further studies should clarify the most appropriate scanning method and the exact place of FDG PET, along with MRI.

FDG PET Imaging of Large-Vessel Vasculitis

Qi Cao and Wengan Chen

Diagnosis of vasculitis is challenging given the nonspecific manifestations of the diseases. [18F]Fluorodeoxyglucose (FDG) positron emission tomography (PET) has been increasingly used for vasculitis in clinic and has been shown to have a potential role in diagnosing large-vessel vasculitis such as giant cell vasculitis and Takayasu vasculitis, in monitoring treatment response, and in predicting disease progression. However, the exact clinical role of FDG PET for vasculitis has not been determined. Diagnosis of vasculitis should not be made solely based on PET. It is also worth noting that FDG PET has limited role in small-size vasculitis, although case reports have shown some success.

Assessment of Therapy Response by FDG PET in Infection and Inflammation

Rakesh Kumar, Sellam Karunanithi, Hongming Zhuang, and Abass Alavi

Positron emission tomography (PET) is a well-known imaging modality in assessing the treatment response to chemotherapy or radiotherapy in various malignancies. A systematic review of the literature reveals a few publications reporting evaluation of the treatment response in benign conditions using PET/computed tomography. PET holds a promising future role in the follow-up of inflammatory or infectious diseases. In this article, [18F]Fluorodeoxyglucose PET as a tool in the evaluation, treatment, and follow-up of infectious and inflammatory diseases is discussed.

Index

PET Clinics

THE CLINICS ARE NOW AVAILABLE ONLINE!

Access your subscription at:
www.theclinics.com

GOAL STATEMENT

The goal of the *PET Clinics* is to keep practicing radiologists and radiology residents up to date with current clinical practice in positron emission tomography by providing timely articles reviewing the state of the art in patient care.

ACCREDITATION

PET Clinics is planned and implemented in accordance with the Essential Areas and Policies of the Accreditation Council for Continuing Medical Education (ACCME) through the joint sponsorship of the University of Virginia School of Medicine and Elsevier. The University of Virginia School of Medicine is accredited by the ACCME to provide continuing medical education for physicians.

The University of Virginia School of Medicine designates this enduring material activity for a maximum of 15 *AMA PRA Category 1 Credit(s)™ for each issue,* 60 credits per year. Physicians should only claim credit commensurate with the extent of their participation in the activity.

The American Medical Association has determined that physicians not licensed in the US who participate in this CME enduring material activity are eligible for a maximum of 15 *AMA PRA Category 1 Credit(s)™* for each issue, 60 credits per year.

Credit can be earned by reading the text material, taking the CME examination online at http://www.theclinics.com/home/cme, and completing the evaluation. After taking the test, you will be required to review any and all incorrect answers. Following completion of the test and evaluation, your credit will be awarded and you may print your certificate.

FACULTY DISCLOSURE/CONFLICT OF INTEREST

The University of Virginia School of Medicine, as an ACCME accredited provider, endorses and strives to comply with the Accreditation Council for Continuing Medical Education (ACCME) Standards of Commercial Support, Commonwealth of Virginia statutes, University of Virginia policies and procedures, and associated federal and private regulations and guidelines on the need for disclosure and monitoring of proprietary and financial interests that may affect the scientific integrity and balance of content delivered in continuing medical education activities under our auspices.

The University of Virginia School of Medicine requires that all CME activities accredited through this institution be developed independently and be scientifically rigorous, balanced and objective in the presentation/discussion of its content, theories and practices.

All authors/editors participating in an accredited CME activity are expected to disclose to the readers relevant financial relationships with commercial entities occurring within the past 12 months (such as grants or research support, employee, consultant, stock holder, member of speakers bureau, etc.). The University of Virginia School of Medicine will employ appropriate mechanisms to resolve potential conflicts of interest to maintain the standards of fair and balanced education to the reader. Questions about specific strategies can be directed to the Office of Continuing Medical Education, University of Virginia School of Medicine, Charlottesville, Virginia.

The faculty and staff of the University of Virginia Office of Continuing Medical Education have no financial affiliations to disclose.

The authors/editors listed below have identified no professional or financial affiliations for themselves or their spouse/partner:

Abass Alavi, MD, PhD (Hon), DSc (Hon) (Consulting and Guest Editor); Sarah Barth, (Acquisitions Editor); Sandip Basu, MBBS (Hons), DRM, DNB, MNAMS; Qi Cao, MD, PhD; Wengen Chen, MD, PhD; Ion Codreanu, MD, PhD; Phyllis Dioguardi, MD, MA; Mohan Doss, PhD, MCCPM; Santosh R. Gaddam, MD; Roland Hustinx, MD, PhD; Sellam Karunanithi, MD; Rakesh Kumar, MD, PhD; Yuejian Liu, MD; Molly Parsons, BA; Patrice Rehm, MD (Test Author); Babak Saboury, MD, MPH; Sabah Servaes, MD; Drew A. Torigian, MD, MA; Bing Xu, MD, PhD; Jigang Yang, MD, PhD; Hongming Zhuang, MD, PhD (Guest Editor); and Pouya Ziai, MD.

The authors/editors listed below identified the following professional or financial affiliations for themselves or their spouse/partner:

Jian Q. Yu, MD, FRCPC is an industry funded research/investigator for Siemens.

Disclosure of Discussion of Non-FDA Approved Uses for Pharmaceutical Products and/or Medical Devices.

The University of Virginia School of Medicine, as an ACCME provider, requires that all faculty presenters identify and disclose any off-label uses for pharmaceutical and medical device products. The University of Virginia School of Medicine recommends that each physician fully review all the available data on new products or procedures prior to clinical use.

TO ENROLL

To enroll in the PET Clinics Continuing Medical Education program, call customer service at 1-800-654-2452 or visit us online at www.theclinics.com/home/cme. The CME program is available to subscribers for an additional fee of $196.00.

Preface
PET Imaging of Infection and Inflammation

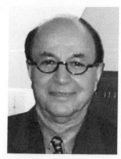 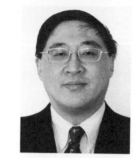

Abass Alavi, MD, PhD (Hon), DSc (Hon)   Hongming Zhuang, MD, PhD
Guest Editors

The introduction of 18F-fluoro-2-deoxglucose (FDG) in 1976 as a joint effort between investigators at the University of Pennsylvania and Brookhaven National Laboratory opened a new era in medical imaging. Although the initial intent of scientists involved in this project was to determine central nervous system function in normal and diseased states, FDG has proven to be of great value in many other domains over the last three decades. Soon after its introduction, FDG was employed to characterize brain tumors, particularly when the differential diagnosis of tumor recurrence versus radiation-induced necrosis was of clinical concern. With the introduction of whole body imaging, numerous malignancies were examined with FDG for accurate diagnosis, staging, response to therapy, and recurrence. In fact, this application has become the most valuable contribution of this agent to the practice of medicine. However, with a wider spread utilization of this methodology, it became apparent that inflammatory reactions due to either underlying infection or autoimmune disorders are readily detected by this technique.

Investigators at various laboratories around the world including those at the University of Pennsylvania have heavily researched the role of FDG-PET in assessing infection and inflammation in a variety of settings. In the past decade, a large number of scientific communications have appeared in the literature, substantiating the role of this very powerful modality in these common disorders.

Attempts have been made to secure reimbursement from Medicare and Medicaid for this particular application. Unfortunately, limited experience in the United States utilizing FDG for this particular domain has resulted in delays of approval. However, in Europe and other countries, FDG is being frequently used for examining patients with a variety of inflammatory reactions. In this issue of the *PET Clinics*, we have updated the current literature on this topic and hope that educating the community of the potential for this very important application of FDG will lead to its future utilization in a clinical setting.

Abass Alavi, MD, PhD (Hon), DSc (Hon)
Division of Nuclear Medicine
Department of Radiology
Hospital of the University of Pennsylvania
3400 Spruce Street
Philadelphia, PA 19104, USA

Hongming Zhuang, MD, PhD
Division of Nuclear Medicine
Department of Radiology
The Children's Hospital of Philadelphia
University of Pennsylvania School of Medicine
34th Street and Civic Center Boulevard
Philadelphia, PA 19104, USA

E-mail addresses:
Abass.Alavi@uphs.upenn.edu (A. Alavi)
zhuanghm@yahoo.com (H. Zhuang)

PET Clin 7 (2012) xi
doi:10.1016/j.cpet.2012.02.001
1556-8598/12/$ – see front matter © 2012 Elsevier Inc. All rights reserved

pet.theclinics.com

Promising Roles of PET in Management of Arthroplasty-Associated Infection

Babak Saboury, MD, MPH[a], Pouya Ziai, MD[a],
Molly Parsons, BA[a], Hongming Zhuang, MD, PhD[b],
Sandip Basu, MBBS (Hons), DRM, DNB, MNAMS[c],
Abass Alavi, MD, PhD (Hon), DSc (Hon)[a],*

KEYWORDS

• Arthroplasty • Infection • Diagnosis • PET/CT • FDG

Joint arthroplasty represents a major innovation in the management of patients with chronic, refractory joint pain. Approximately 700,000 total hip arthroplasties (THA) and total knee arthroplasties (TKA) are done yearly in the United States.[1] Considering the increasing size of the aging population as well as the obesity epidemic ongoing in this country and many others around the world, this number is predicted to go up even further in the future. THA and TKA have been successful in reducing pain and improving the quality of life of patients with hip and knee pathologic conditions. Unfortunately, however, a subset of these patients will go on to experience persistent hip and knee pain following their initial intervention leading to continued patient suffering, frustration, and the potential need for revision surgery.

Aseptic loosening and periprosthetic infection are 2 of the most common reasons for joint pain following arthroplasty.[2] Infection of a total joint replacement is among the most feared complications in lower limb arthroplasties.[3,4] The infection rate is 1% to 4% for primary lower limb arthroplasties and can exceed 30% after revision arthroplasty.[4] It usually requires the extirpation of the prosthesis and cement, long-term intravenous antibiotic therapy, and eventual reimplantation of a new device at a later operation. In addition, if patients have persistent infection at the time of intended reimplantation, further debridement instead of a joint replacement is required. In contrast, an aseptic process manifesting as a failed joint arthroplasty requires limited diagnostic studies to determine the cause of loosening followed by the removal of the original loose prosthesis and reimplantation during a single surgical procedure.[5] Aseptic loosening is responsible for failure in nearly 90% of complicated cases. The rate of aseptic loosening varies with prosthetic design, prosthetic implantation technique, and wear debris. This clear-cut difference in planning for the management of these 2 complications emphasizes the importance of preoperative identification of the underlying process.

The diagnostic algorithms for the evaluation of painful arthroplasties are often complex and challenging. Unfortunately, despite these complex algorithms, the differentiation between the 2 most common types of failure remains difficult. The accurate diagnosis of an infected implant can be made from the clinical history and physical examination in only about 25% of patients because

[a] Department of Radiology, School of Medicine, University of Pennsylvania, 3400 Spruce Street, Philadelphia, PA 19104, USA
[b] Division of Nuclear Medicine, Department of Radiology, The Children's Hospital of Philadelphia, University of Pennsylvania School of Medicine, 34th Street and Civic Center Boulevard, Philadelphia, PA 19104, USA
[c] Radiation Medicine Centre, Bhabha Atomic Research Centre, Tata Memorial Hospital Annexe, Parel, Bombay 400012, India
* Corresponding author.
E-mail address: Abass.Alavi@uphs.upenn.edu

PET Clin 7 (2012) 139–150
doi:10.1016/j.cpet.2012.01.002
1556-8598/12/$ – see front matter © 2012 Published by Elsevier Inc.

many of the signs and symptoms of infection can overlap with other clinical conditions, such as aseptic loosening, intra-articular hematoma, and instability.

In most cases, significant additional diagnostic testing is required to establish the diagnosis.[6] Inflammatory markers, such as erythrocyte sedimentation rate and C-reactive protein level, are nonspecific. These markers are elevated in both cases of periprosthetic infection and aseptic loosening.[7] Joint aspiration has been reported to approach a specificity of 100%; however, the wide range of reported sensitivity (0%–100%) by different research groups has made it an unreliable diagnostic modality in differentiating septic and aseptic prosthesis loosening.[8] In addition, the aspiration of the joint is invasive, and the contamination of a noninfected joint is always a major concern. Plain radiography lacks the preferred sensitivity and specificity for an ideal diagnostic test, and cross-sectional imaging modalities, such as computed tomography and magnetic resonance imaging are distorted by artifacts produced by the metal implants. Radionuclide imaging, reflecting physiologic rather than anatomic changes, is less affected by the presence of metallic implants and represents an attractive alternative for the evaluation of periprosthetic infection. Many consider combined leukocyte–marrow scintigraphy the imaging gold standard in diagnosing prosthetic joint infection. However, there are drawbacks to this imaging technique, including it being labor intensive, expensive, not widely available, and time consuming, as well as the associated risk of handling blood products[9] and the lack of accuracy (**Figs. 1** and **2**). As such, the best preoperative diagnostic strategy is yet to be determined.

Fluorodeoxyglucose positron emission tomography (FDG-PET) imaging is a useful imaging technique for the detection of both infectious and inflammatory processes. Many reports have noted the affinity of FDG for active inflammatory and infectious disorders,[10] such as sarcoidosis,[11–13] the abdominal abscess,[14] brain abscess,[15] lung abscess,[16] renal abscess,[17] inflammatory pancreatic disease,[18] lobar pneumonia,[19,20] asthma,[21] tuberculosis,[22,23] colitis,[24] sinusitis,[25] myositis,[26] mastitis,[27] vasculitis,[28,29] deep venous thrombosis,[30] and thyroiditis.[31] In addition to this wide range of applications, FDG-PET imaging has also been used for detecting infections in orthopedic patients.[32,33] The established niche of FDG-PET in the diagnosis of infectious disorders and the developing role of this modality in the diagnosis of complicated orthopedic conditions make this a likely investigative and management tool for patients with complicated prosthetic implants. The following review of the literature is meant to clearly delineate the current status of FDG-PET and FDG-PET/computed tomography (CT) in the diagnosis and management of arthroplasty-associated infections (**Tables 1** and **2**).

USE OF [18]FDG-PET IN THE DIAGNOSIS OF ENDOPROSTHETIC LOOSENING OF KNEE AND HIP IMPLANTS

FDG-PET imaging has been applied extensively for the diagnosis of periprosthetic infection of the hip and knee. An early investigation by Zhuang and colleagues[34] in 2001 was one of the first to examine the feasibility of FDG-PET in the diagnosis of lower limb periprosthetic infection. They prospectively evaluated 62 patients (74 prosthesis) with a painful lower limb who had undergone hip (38) and knee arthroplasty (36). FDG-PET was considered positive for infection when there was an increased intensity of uptake at the bone-prosthesis interface (FDG uptake limited to the soft tissues adjacent to the neck of prosthesis was not considered a sign of infection). The result of their study showed a promising role for FDG-PET imaging in diagnosing (specificity of 89.3% and 72.0% for hip and knee respectively) and excluding (sensitivity of 90.0% and 90.9%

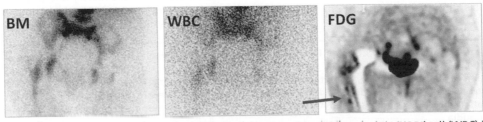

Fig. 1. In this patient with suspected prosthesis infection, bone marrow (BM) and white blood cell (WBC) imaging show identical patterns which was interpreted to exclude infection. However, FDG-PET reveal intense uptake in the lateral aspect of proximal femur in the interface between prosthesis and bone (*red arrow*). This finding was interpreted to represent infection, which was confirmed by further investigation.

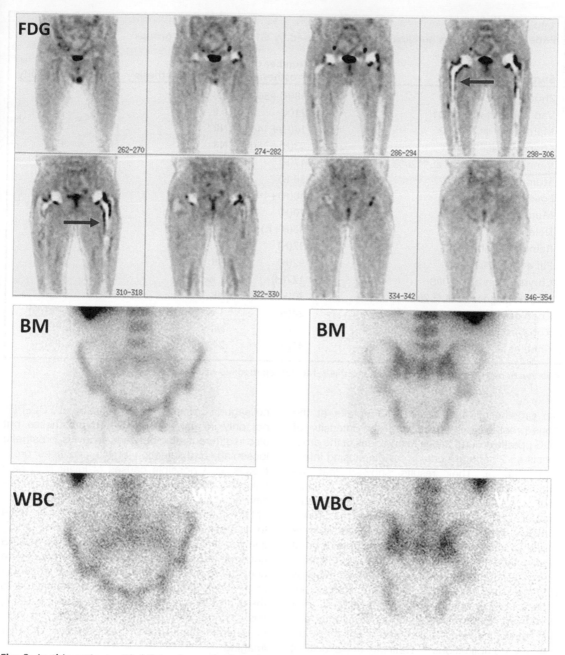

Fig. 2. In this patient with bilateral prosthesis and suspected infection in both sides, FDG-PET images reveal a pattern suggestive of infection in both sides (*red arrows*), which was confirmed by further assessment. However, bone marrow (BM) and white blood cell (WBC) images reveal identical patterns that were interpreted to be false negative in this patient with proven infection.

for hip and knee respectively) hip and knee prosthesis infection. Their study also emphasized that the location of the uptake at the bone-prosthesis interface and not just the intensity of uptake is critically important in diagnosing infection in this patient population.

One of the difficulties in diagnostic imaging in general is creating a universal assessment scheme

that can be adapted by radiologists in different clinical settings and with varying level of expertise. Accurate identification of periprosthetic infections is no exception and necessitates a validated set of diagnostic criteria. The same group went on to confirm their prior findings and further highlight the importance of the location of FDG uptake in diagnosing periprosthetic infection. Evaluating 41

Table 1
Patient characteristics and imaging methods used by different research groups

Study and Year	Number of Patients	Number of Prosthesis	Age of Prosthesis	Tracer	Modality
Zhuang et al,[34] 2001	62	38(H)+36(K)	0.6–9 y	FDG	PET
Van Acker et al,[39] 2001	21	21(K)	0.6–9 y	FDG	PET
Manthey et al,[38] 2002	23	14(H)+14(K)	NR	FDG	PET
Chacko et al,[37] 2003	NR	53(H)+36(K)	NR	FDG	PET
Vanquickenborne et al,[40] 2003	17	17(H)	0.2–13.6 y	FDG	PET
Stumpe et al,[44] 2004	35	36(H)	1–21.6 y	FDG	PET
Love et al,[42] 2004	59	40(H)+19(K)	1 w–20 y	FDG	PET
Mumme et al,[45] 2005	50	70(H)	1–31 y	FDG	PET
Delank et al,[46] 2006	26	36(H+K)	0.8–19.4 y	FDG	PET
Reinartz et al,[43] 2005	63	92(H)	1–31 y	FDG	PET
Pill et al,[41] 2006	89	92(H)	NR	FDG	PET
Chryssikos et al,[47] 2008	113	127(H)	1 w–20 y	FDG	PET
Mayer-Wagner et al,[48] 2010	32	30(H)+44(K)	NR	FDG	PET
Chen et al,[49] 2010	24	24(H)	1 w–20.5 y	FDG	PET/CT
Kobayashi et al,[50] 2011	49	65(H)	NR	18F-NaF	PET
Choe et al,[51] 2011	40	46(H)	2–28 y	18F-NaF	PET

Abbreviations: H, hip prosthesis; K, knee prosthesis; NR, not reported; w, week; y, year.

hip prostheses, they used FDG uptake at the bone-prosthesis interface and the intensity of FDG uptake around the head and neck of the prosthesis as 2 separate criteria for diagnosing infection (**Fig. 3**). Their results showed that the intensity of uptake was on average 2 to 3 times less in patients with infection but was consistently located at the bone-prosthesis interface. Those patients with an uncomplicated prosthesis were found to have a greater intensity of uptake but it was located around the head and neck of the prosthesis (ie, not near the bone).[35] As described by Zhuang and colleagues,[34] the nonspecific increase in FDG uptake around the head or neck portion of the prosthesis occurs frequently and can persist for many years, even in patients without any complications.[36] Defining these distinct uptake patterns illustrates that the site of tracer accumulation is essential in the accurate diagnosis of postarthroplasty hip infection and will aide in minimizing false positive results in the future.

Chacko and colleagues[37] compared the effectiveness of FDG-PET in the diagnosis of hip and knee prosthesis infection. They reported equal sensitivity of FDG-PET in detecting hip and knee periprosthetic infection (91.7% and 92.0% respectively); however, specificity was shown to be higher in hip arthroplasty cases compared with knee cases. Looking to further expand the diagnostic capabilities of FDG-PET, Manthey and

colleagues[38] described the efficacy of FDG-PET not only in diagnosing infected prostheses but also in differentiating between synovitis, prosthetic loosening, and infection of hip and knee prostheses as 3 possible causes of lower limb pain following arthroplasty. They included both intensity and location of periprosthetic radiotracer uptake in their analysis. A visual quantitative scale to differentiate septic and aseptic loosening showed that high and intermediate levels of FDG uptakes at the bone-prosthesis interface were considered positive for infection and loosening respectively. Any amount of uptake restricted to the synovium was interpreted as synovitis. Using this method, they reported an accuracy of 96% in differentiating these 3 entities by FDG-PET imaging.

The introduction of a new imaging modality as a potential diagnostic tool requires vigorous testing and validation, particularly against those modalities currently being used. As previously mentioned, combined leukocyte-marrow scintigraphy had become one of the predominant imaging modalities used by clinicians in diagnosing periprosthetic infection. As the role of FDG-PET in diagnosing complicated prostheses began to show more promise, a comparison of these 2 studies was essential in establishing the best standard of care for these patients. Comparing FDG-PET with combined leukocyte-marrow scintigraphy in 21

Table 2
FDG PET image interpretation methods and results

Study and Year	Criteria for Positivity	Sensitivity (%)	Specificity (%)
Zhuang et al,[34] 2001	Increased FDG uptake at the BPI (uptake limited to the soft tissues adjacent to the neck or the tip of the femoral component was not considered a sign of infection)	90.5	81.1
Van Acker et al,[39] 2001	Increased FDG uptake at the BPI	100	73.3
Manthey et al,[38] 2002	Increased FDG uptake at the BPI	100	100
Chacko et al,[37] 2003	Increased FDG uptake at the BPI (uptake limited to the soft tissues adjacent to the neck or the tip of the femoral component was not considered a sign of infection)	91.7	89.2
Vanquickenborne et al,[40] 2003	FDG uptake of grade 2 or higher and different from control group	87.5	77.8
Stumpe et al,[44] 2004	Diffuse increase of FDG uptake of grade 3 or higher along the BPI	33.3	80.8
Love et al,[42] 2004	Criteria1: Any periprosthetic activity regardless of location and intensity	100	9
	Criteria 2: Any periprosthetic activity regardless of location and intensity + no corresponding activity in the marrow image	96	35
	Criteria 3: Increased FDG uptake at the BPI regardless of intensity	52	34
	Criteria 4: Semiquantitative analysis (TBR threshold of 3.6 and 3.9 for hip and knee, respectively)	36	97
Mumme et al,[45] 2005	Increased FDG uptake at BPI and in the periprosthetic soft tissue	91	92
Delank et al,[46] 2006	Increased FDG uptake in the periprosthetic soft tissue	40	100
Reinartz et al,[43] 2005	Increased FDG uptake in the periprosthetic soft tissue	93.9	94.9
Pill et al,[41] 2006	Increased FDG uptake at the BPI (uptake limited to the soft tissues adjacent to the neck or the tip of the femoral component was not considered a sign of infection)	95.2	93.0
Chryssikos et al,[47] 2008	Increased FDG uptake at the BPI (uptake limited to the soft tissues adjacent to the neck or the tip of the femoral component was not considered a sign of infection)	84.9	92.6
Mayer-Wagner et al,[48] 2010	Increased FDG uptake at the BPI + intensity of FDG uptake	80	87
Chen et al,[49] 2010	Increased FDG uptake at the BPI (uptake limited to the soft tissues adjacent to the neck or the tip of the femoral component was not considered a sign of infection)	100	75
Kobayashi et al,[50] 2011	Significant 18-F fluoride uptake through more than half of the BPI	95	98

Abbreviations: BPI, bone-prosthesis interface; TBR, target-to-background ratio.

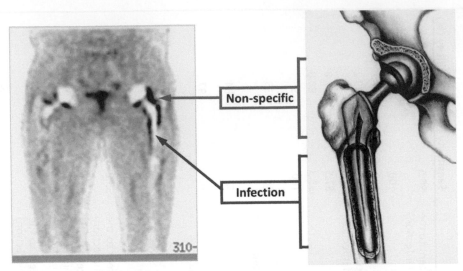

Fig. 3. Right panel: regions of FDG uptake corresponding to the site of nonspecific aseptic reaction and infection are shown in this diagram. Left panel: coronal image of a patient with bilateral painful hip prostheses. Focal uptake is noted around the neck region of prosthesis (*blue arrow*). There is also an intense uptake in the proximal upper femur in the interface between prosthesis and bone (*red arrow*), which represents infection (confirmed by further investigation). (*From* Chacko TK, Zhuang H, Stevenson K, et al. The importance of the location of fluorodeoxyglucose uptake in periprosthetic infection in painful hip prostheses. Nucl Med Commun 2002;23:851–5; with permission.)

patients with painful knee prosthesis, Van Acker and colleagues[39] reported a high sensitivity but insufficient specificity of FDG-PET for the detection of metallic implant infection (**Fig. 4**). Both methods were reported to have a sensitivity of 100%; however, specificity was shown to be 73% and 93% for FDG-PET and combined leukocyte-marrow scintigraphy respectively.

Several research teams have further examined the comparative relationship between FDG-PET and combined leukocyte-marrow scintigraphy. In a study of 17 symptomatic patients with hip arthroplasty, Vanquickenborne and colleagues[40] showed that FDG-PET alone has the same sensitivity as conventional combined leukocyte-marrow scintigraphy in detecting periprosthetic hip infection; however, the specificity was shown to be suboptimal compared with those of combined leukocyte-marrow scintigraphy, 77.8% and 100%. The investigators attribute this difference in specificity to increased FDG uptake seen in cases of noninfectious inflammation. In a similar study, Pill and colleagues[41] also compared the accuracy of FDG-PET and combined leukocyte-marrow scintigraphy in diagnosing periprosthetic infection. Investigating 89 patients for the revision of painful hip prosthesis, they reported a comparable specificity (93.0% and 95.1% respectively)

A   **B**

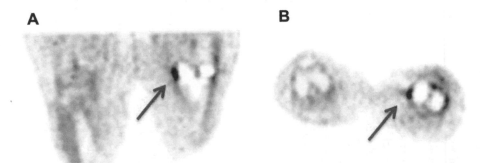

Fig. 4. Image (*A*) (coronal section) and image (*B*) (transaxial section) of an FDG-PET scan of a patient with left knee prosthesis demonstrate a focus of intense FDG uptake in the medial aspect of femoral component of prosthesis at the bone-prosthesis interface (*arrows*). Operative findings and histopathology confirmed the presence of infection.

of these 2 techniques. However, FDG-PET was shown to have a substantially higher sensitivity of 95.2% compared with 50.0% for combined leukocyte-marrow scintigraphy. In a study including 59 patients with failed hip (40) and knee (19) arthroplasties, Love and colleagues[42] evaluated FDG uptake using a coincidence detection system. Their study showed that even by using the most favorable schemes, the best accuracy of FDG-PET was 71% for the detection of infection, which was much lower than the 95% accuracy of combined leukocyte-marrow scintigraphy in their study population. However, the results of this study may be limited by the use of a coincidence detection system rather than a dedicated PET system.

Another imaging study that has been used in the setting of prosthetic complications is triple-phase bone scintigraphy (TPBS) and, thus, a comparison with FDG-PET was warranted. In a study by Reinartz and colleagues,[43] FDG-PET was shown to have much greater capability in detecting complications following hip arthroplasty than TPBS. They evaluated 92 hip prostheses in patients presenting with increasing pain in the region of the arthroplasty. Regarding the ability to differentiate between loosening and infection, FDG-PET achieved sensitivity, specificity, and accuracy of 93.9%, 94.9%, and 94.6%, respectively, whereas values of 68%, 76%, and 74% were achieved by TPBS. They confirmed that FDG uptake of the acetabular and proximal aspect of the femoral component of hip replacements does not represent a sign of infection (**Fig. 5**). They also concluded that the intensity of the FDG uptake alone is misleading and cannot be used to interpret postarthroplasty complications. These findings not only emphasis the improved

sensitivity, specificity, and accuracy afforded by FDG-PET over TPBS but they also provide further support for the importance of location rather than intensity of FDG uptake in the diagnosis of periprosthetic infection.

Comparing the diagnostic efficacy of FDG-PET, conventional radiography, and TPBS in differentiating septic and aseptic loosening of hip prostheses, Stumpe and colleagues[44] found a similar performance of FDG-PET and TPBS. However, FDG-PET was shown to be more specific but less sensitive than conventional radiography in diagnosing periprosthetic hip infection. The average sensitivities and specificities of 2 readers for the 3 tests, FDG-PET, conventional radiography, and TPBS, were 27.5%, 83.5%, 50.0% and 83.0%, 57.5%, 90.0%, respectively. This finding argues for the use of FDG-PET in patients with a high pretest suspicion of infection but for which confirmation is desired before surgical intervention.

Mumme and colleagues[45] compared the diagnostic potential of FDG-PET and TPBS for differentiating septic and aseptic loosening of hip prostheses. Evaluating 50 patients with clinical signs of arthroplastic loosening, they reported higher sensitivity, specificity, and accuracy for FDG-PET than TPBS with technetium 99m hydroxyethylene diphosphonate (99mTc-HDP). There was a significant correlation between FDG-PET interpretation and intraoperative histologic findings. They also concluded that standardized uptake value (SUV) measurement is not a reliable measurement in differentiating septic and aseptic loosening and should not be used as the only criteria in this context.

In a study by Delank and colleagues,[46] they concluded that FDG-PET is a reliable method to

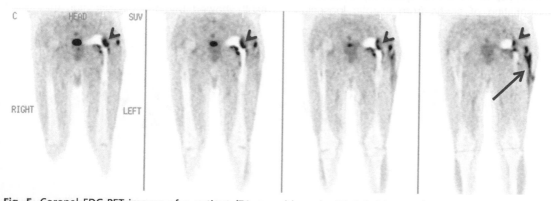

Fig. 5. Coronal FDG-PET images of a patient (71-year-old man) with left hip prosthesis and left lateral thigh abscess. Arrowheads show mild FDG uptake in the proximal compartment of the left hip prosthesis secondary to aseptic inflammatory reaction. Increased uptake in the left lateral thigh (*arrow*) is caused by an abscess in soft tissue of the upper lateral thigh (absence of infected prosthesis confirmed by long-term clinical follow-up).

detect periprosthetic inflammation of the knee and hip but there is no role for this modality in differentiating between septic and aseptic periprosthetic inflammation. Evaluating 21 patients planned for prosthetic loosening revision surgery with FDG-PET, they reported a sensitivity of 100% and 45.5% for septic and aseptic loosening of lower limb arthroplasty respectively. Reliable differentiation between these 2 diagnoses was not possible using this method. The limited number of study participants in many of these studies limited the power of the results and, thus, made it abundantly clear that there was a definite need for a larger-scale study.

In contrast, however, Chryssikos and colleagues[47] reported excellent accuracy of FDG-PET in differentiating septic from aseptic painful hip prosthesis in a larger, prospective, multicenter study on 113 patients. Considering increased FDG uptake at the prosthesis-bone interface suggestive of infection (**Fig. 6**), they were able to correctly detect 28 of 33 infected cases (sensitivity 84.8%) and to rule out infection in 87 of the 94 aseptic hips (specificity 92.6%).

A study by Mayer-Wagner and colleagues[48] looked at the role of [18]FDG-PET in differentiating stable prostheses, aseptic loosening, and septic loosening in both hip and knee arthroplasties using strict interpretation criteria. They found that [18]FDG-PET was a worthwhile preoperative modality for the detection of hip prosthesis stability versus loosening with a sensitivity and specificity of 80% and 87% respectively. However, the study had only intermediated results for the diagnosis of prosthetic infection with a sensitivity of 75% and specificity of 71%. The results were less conclusive regarding the diagnosis of knee prosthesis loosening and infection. A sensitivity of 56% and specificity of 82% for diagnosing loosening and a sensitivity of 14% and specificity of 82% for differentiating of septic from aseptic loosening

following total knee arthroplasty were reported in the study. Therefore, although [18]FDG-PET seems to be a valuable diagnostic tool in the evaluation of complicated hip prosthesis, further work and the development of better diagnostic criteria needs to be conducted to implement this method in patients with complicated TKA.

In a pilot study, Chen and colleagues evaluated the utility of FDG-PET/CT in detecting latent infection at the site of an interim hip spacer following the resection of an infected hip prosthesis.[49] They evaluated 24 patients, 12 with an interim hip spacer and 12 with a primary symptomatic hip prosthesis as controls. To compare diagnostic accuracy, they analyzed both nonattenuation corrected (NAC) and attenuation corrected PET/CT images. Using the criteria proposed by Chacko and colleagues,[37] they reported a sensitivity of 100% for FDG PET/CT in detecting infection in both patient groups; however, specificity was reported to be 50.0% and 62.5% in the interim spacer group and primary arthroplasty group respectively. When NAC images were used, these values improved to 62.5% and 87.5% respectively.[49]

USE OF F-18 FLUORIDE PET IN THE DIAGNOSIS OF ENDOPROSTHETIC LOOSENING OF HIP IMPLANTS

In a novel study by Kobayashi and colleagues,[50] they described the effectiveness of F-18 fluoride PET imaging in differentiating septic from aseptic prosthesis loosening after THA. Prospectively they evaluated 65 joints after THA comprised of 27 asymptomatic (control), 11 symptomatic treated conservatively, and 27 symptomatic treated surgically. Based on the amount of bone-prosthesis interface radiotracer uptake, they classified PET imaging into 3 types (**Fig. 7**). Their result showed that the classification they used

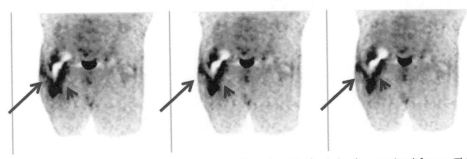

Fig. 6. Coronal images reveal intense uptake surrounding the prosthesis in the proximal femur. This finding is suggestive of infection, which was proven by further investigation (*arrowhead*). In addition, there is evidence of a fistula tract connecting to the sites of femoral infection to the soft tissues of the lateral aspect of the upper thigh (*arrow*).

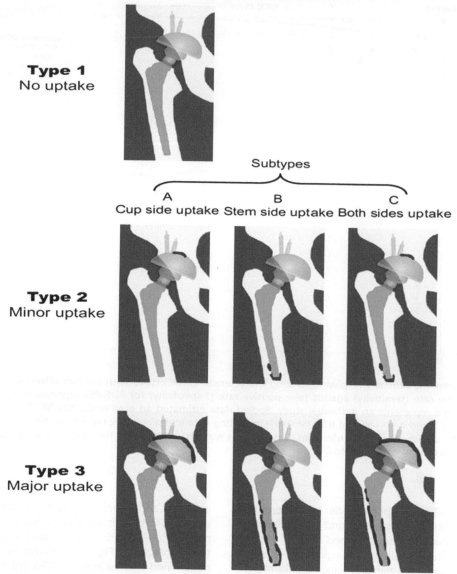

Type 1
No uptake

Subtypes

A   B   C
Cup side uptake Stem side uptake Both sides uptake

Type 2
Minor uptake

Type 3
Major uptake

Fig. 7. The classification of F-18 fluoride PET uptake patterns in patients with THA. In type 1 uptake there is no uptake around the implant. In type 2 there is a minor level of uptake that is localized within one-half of the bone-implant interface. In type 3 there is a significant uptake spreading through more than half of the bone-implant interface. There are also subtypes for type 2 and 3: (A) uptake localized on the cup side, (B) localized at the stem side, and (C) localized on both the cup and stem sides. (*Reprinted from* Kobayashi N, Inaba Y, Choe H, et al. Use of F-18 Fluoride PET to differentiate septic from aseptic loosening in total hip arthroplasty patients. Clin Nucl Med 2011;36(11):e156–61; with permission; see **Fig. 1.**)

was significantly associated with the final diagnosis because the type 3 uptake pattern had the sensitivity and specificity of 95% and 98% respectively for the diagnosis of infection. Using SUVmax, they also reported a significant difference between SUVmax of septic and aseptic loosening because it was significantly higher in symptomatic patients than controls and was also significantly higher in septic joints compared with those that were not infected.

Choe and colleagues[51] used F-18 fluoride PET scanning in the preoperative planning of 23 patients scheduled for THA revision surgery. They used the images to semiquantitatively determine those areas of the joint with the most F-18 fluoride uptake either on the acetabular or femoral side of the prosthesis. The investigators proceeded to use these 2 locations for sampling for histopathologic examination, microbiological culture, and real-time polymerase chain reaction.

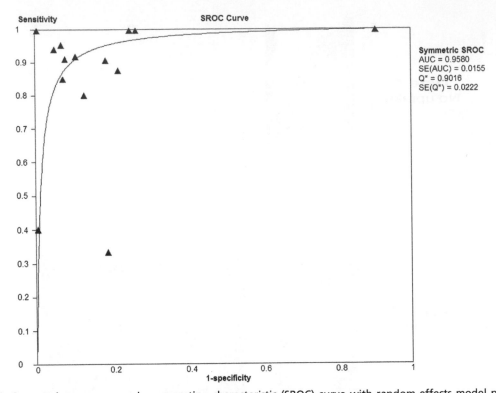

Fig. 8. Symmetric summary receiver operating characteristic (SROC) curve with random effects model plotting true positive rate (sensitivity) against false positive rate (1-specificity) for FDG-PET reported in the literature. Each triangle represents an individual study. Pooled data estimated an area under the SROC curve (AUC) of 0.96 (SE: 0.02) and a Q* value of 0.90 (SE: 0.02) indicating excellent diagnostic capabilities for FDG-PET in diagnosing arthroplasty-associated infections. Data analysis was performed using the publically available dedicated meta-analysis software tool Meta-DiSc version 1.4.[52]

They classified 17 patients as having areas of major uptake before surgery, and a definitive diagnosis of infection was confirmed in all 17 of these patients. The remaining 6 surgical patients had preoperative scans with only minor-uptake regions and were found to be aseptic when the acetabular and femoral spaces were sampled. A control group had no regions of major uptake and only 3 regions of mild uptake. Although the sample size was small, these data illustrate the potential role of F-18 PET imaging in perioperative planning in patients with complicated prostheses to ensure optimal tissue sampling and a reduction in false negative results.

Discussion

The diagnostic dilemma faced by orthopedic surgeons when faced with patients with a complicated prosthetic implant is ongoing. The current imaging modalities being used include plain film, combined leukocyte-marrow scintigraphy, and TPBS, yet no one method has proved to be highly sensitive and specific as well as safe and time effective. Research has shown that there is a definite role for FDG-PET in the diagnosis of periprosthetic infection (**Fig. 8**). Several studies have determined and verified the FDG uptake patterns essential for diagnosis as well as the improved sensitivity and specificity of this method compared with the more traditional modalities. Proper diagnosis of prosthetic infection has a huge clinical impact for both the clinician and patients in terms of individualized perioperative treatment planning. An accurate diagnosis before revision surgery allows the physician to better anticipate intraoperative and postoperative complications and predict recovery time. Further prospective research in FDG-PET imaging in periprosthetic infection is necessary to validate this approach and advances its current utility.

ACKNOWLEDGMENTS

We acknowledge Björn Blomberg for his contribution.

REFERENCES

1. Love C, Marwin SE, Palestro CJ. Nuclear medicine and the infected joint replacement. Semin Nucl Med 2009;39(1):66–78.

2. Clohisy JC, Calvert G, Tull F, et al. Reasons for revision hip surgery: a retrospective review. Clin Orthop Relat Res 2004;(429):188–92.

3. Andrews HJ, Arden GP, Hart GM, et al. Deep infection after total hip replacement. J Bone Joint Surg Br 1981;63-B(1):53–7.

4. Maderazo EG, Judson S, Pasternak H. Late infections of total joint prostheses. A review and recommendations for prevention. Clin Orthop Relat Res 1988;(229):131–42.

5. Rand JA, Morrey BF, Bryan RS. Management of the infected total joint arthroplasty. Orthop Clin North Am 1984;15(3):491–504.

6. Fitzgerald RH Jr. Diagnosis and management of the infected hip prosthesis. Orthopedics 1995;18(9): 833–5.

7. Spangehl MJ, Masri BA, O'Connell JX, et al. Prospective analysis of preoperative and intraoperative investigations for the diagnosis of infection at the sites of two hundred and two revision total hip arthroplasties. J Bone Joint Surg Am 1999;81(5):672–83.

8. Barrack RL, Jennings RW, Wolfe MW, et al. The Coventry Award. The value of preoperative aspiration before total knee revision. Clin Orthop Relat Res 1997;(345):8–16.

9. Reinartz P. FDG-PET in patients with painful hip and knee arthroplasty: technical breakthrough or just more of the same. Q J Nucl Med Mol Imaging 2009;53(1):41–50.

10. Alavi A, Buchpiguel CA, Loessner A. Is there a role for FDG PET imaging in the management of patients with sarcoidosis? J Nucl Med 1994;35(10):1650–2.

11. Lewis PJ, Salama A. Uptake of fluorine-18-fluorodeoxyglucose in sarcoidosis. J Nucl Med 1994; 35(10):1647–9.

12. Yamada Y, Uchida Y, Tatsumi K, et al. Fluorine-18-fluorodeoxyglucose and carbon-11-methionine evaluation of lymphadenopathy in sarcoidosis. J Nucl Med 1998;39(7):1160–6.

13. Yasuda S, Shohtsu A, Ide M, et al. High fluorine-18 labeled deoxyglucose uptake in sarcoidosis. Clin Nucl Med 1996;21(12):983–4.

14. Tahara T, Ichiya Y, Kuwabara Y, et al. High [18F]-fluorodeoxyglucose uptake in abdominal abscesses: a PET study. J Comput Assist Tomogr 1989;13(5): 829–31.

15. Meyer MA, Frey KA, Schwaiger M. Discordance between F-18 fluorodeoxyglucose uptake and contrast enhancement in a brain abscess. Clin Nucl Med 1993;18(8):682–4.

16. Yen RF, Chen ML, Liu FY, et al. False-positive 2-[F-18]-fluoro-2-deoxy-D-glucose positron emission tomography studies for evaluation of focal pulmonary abnormalities. J Formos Med Assoc 1998; 97(9):642–5.

17. Kaya Z, Kotzerke J, Keller F. FDG PET diagnosis of septic kidney in a renal transplant patient. Transpl Int 1999;12(2):156.

18. Shreve PD. Focal fluorine-18 fluorodeoxyglucose accumulation in inflammatory pancreatic disease. Eur J Nucl Med 1998;25(3):259–64.

19. Kapucu LO, Meltzer CC, Townsend DW, et al. Fluorine-18-fluorodeoxyglucose uptake in pneumonia. J Nucl Med 1998;39(7):1267–9.

20. Jones HA, Sriskandan S, Peters AM, et al. Dissociation of neutrophil emigration and metabolic activity in lobar pneumonia and bronchiectasis. Eur Respir J 1997;10(4):795–803.

21. Taylor IK, Hill AA, Hayes M, et al. Imaging allergen-invoked airway inflammation in atopic asthma with [18F]-fluorodeoxyglucose and positron emission tomography. Lancet 1996;347(9006):937–40.

22. Patz EF Jr, Lowe VJ, Hoffman JM, et al. Focal pulmonary abnormalities: evaluation with F-18 fluorodeoxyglucose PET scanning. Radiology 1993;188(2): 487–90.

23. Bakheet SM, Powe J, Ezzat A, et al. F-18-FDG uptake in tuberculosis. Clin Nucl Med 1998;23(11): 739–42.

24. Hannah A, Scott AM, Akhurst T, et al. Abnormal colonic accumulation of fluorine-18-FDG in pseudomembranous colitis. J Nucl Med 1996;37(10):1683–5.

25. Yasuda S, Shohtsu A, Ide M, et al. Elevated F-18 FDG uptake in plasmacyte-rich chronic maxillary sinusitis. Clin Nucl Med 1998;23(3):176–8.

26. Gysen M, Stroobants S, Mortelmans L. Proliferative myositis: a case of a pseudomalignant process. Clin Nucl Med 1998;23(12):836–8.

27. Bakheet SM, Powe J, Kandil A, et al. F-18 FDG uptake in breast infection and inflammation. Clin Nucl Med 2000;25(2):100–3.

28. De Winter F, Petrovic M, Van de Wiele C, et al. Imaging of giant cell arteritis: evidence of splenic involvement using FDG positron emission tomography. Clin Nucl Med 2000;25(8):633–4.

29. Hara M, Goodman PC, Leder RA. FDG-PET finding in early-phase Takayasu arteritis. J Comput Assist Tomogr 1999;23(1):16–8.

30. Chang KJ, Zhuang H, Alavi A. Detection of chronic recurrent lower extremity deep venous thrombosis on fluorine-18 fluorodeoxyglucose positron emission tomography. Clin Nucl Med 2000;25(10):838–9.

31. Yasuda S, Shohsu A, Ide M, et al. Diffuse F-18 FDG uptake in chronic thyroiditis. Clin Nucl Med 1997; 22(5):341.

32. Guhlmann A, Brecht-Krauss D, Suger G, et al. Chronic osteomyelitis: detection with FDG PET and correlation with histopathologic findings. Radiology 1998;206(3):749–54.

33. Sugawara Y, Braun DK, Kison PV, et al. Rapid detection of human infections with fluorine-18 fluorodeoxyglucose and positron emission tomography: preliminary results. Eur J Nucl Med 1998;25(9):1238–43.

34. Zhuang H, Duarte PS, Pourdehnad M, et al. The promising role of 18F-FDG PET in detecting infected lower limb prosthesis implants. J Nucl Med 2001; 42(1):44–8.

35. Chacko TK, Zhuang H, Stevenson K, et al. The importance of the location of fluorodeoxyglucose uptake in periprosthetic infection in painful hip prostheses. Nucl Med Commun 2002;23(9):851–5.

36. Zhuang H, Chacko TK, Hickeson M, et al. Persistent non-specific FDG uptake on PET imaging following hip arthroplasty. Eur J Nucl Med Mol Imaging 2002; 29(10):1328–33.

37. Chacko TK, Zhuang H, Nakhoda KZ, et al. Applications of fluorodeoxyglucose positron emission tomography in the diagnosis of infection. Nucl Med Commun 2003;24(6):615–24.

38. Manthey N, Reinhard P, Moog F, et al. The use of [18 F]fluorodeoxyglucose positron emission tomography to differentiate between synovitis, loosening and infection of hip and knee prostheses. Nucl Med Commun 2002;23(7):645–53.

39. Van Acker F, Nuyts J, Maes A, et al. FDG-PET, 99mtc-HMPAO white blood cell SPET and bone scintigraphy in the evaluation of painful total knee arthroplasti. Eur J Nucl Med 2001;28(10):1496–504.

40. Vanquickenborne B, Maes A, Nuyts J, et al. The value of (18)FDG-PET for the detection of infected hip prosthesis. Eur J Nucl Med Mol Imaging 2003; 30(5):705–15.

41. Pill SG, Parvizi J, Tang PH, et al. Comparison of fluorodeoxyglucose positron emission tomography and (111)indium-white blood cell imaging in the diagnosis of periprosthetic infection of the hip. J Arthroplasty 2006;21(6 Suppl 2):91–7.

42. Love C, Marwin SE, Tomas MB, et al. Diagnosing infection in the failed joint replacement: a comparison of coincidence detection 18F-FDG and 111In-labeled leukocyte/99mTc-sulfur colloid marrow imaging. J Nucl Med 2004;45(11):1864–71.

43. Reinartz P, Mumme T, Hermanns B, et al. Radionuclide imaging of the painful hip arthroplasty: positron-emission tomography versus triple-phase bone scanning. J Bone Joint Surg Br 2005;87(4):465–70.

44. Stumpe KD, Nötzli HP, Zanetti M, et al. FDG PET for differentiation of infection and aseptic loosening in total hip replacements: comparison with conventional radiography and three-phase bone scintigraphy. Radiology 2004;231(2):333–41.

45. Mumme T, Reinartz P, Alfer J, et al. Diagnostic values of positron emission tomography versus triple-phase bone scan in hip arthroplasty loosening. Arch Orthop Trauma Surg 2005;125(5):322–9.

46. Delank KS, Schmidt M, Michael JW, et al. The implications of 18F-FDG PET for the diagnosis of endoprosthetic loosening and infection in hip and knee arthroplasty: results from a prospective, blinded study. BMC 2006;7:20.

47. Chryssikos T, Parvizi J, Ghanem E, et al. FDG-PET imaging can diagnose periprosthetic infection of the hip. Clin Orthop Relat Res 2008;466(6):1338–42.

48. Mayer-Wagner S, Mayer W, Maegerlein S, et al. Use of 18F-FDG-PET in the diagnosis of endoprosthetic loosening of knee and hip implants. Arch Orthop Trauma Surg 2010;130(10):1231–8.

49. Chen SH, Ho KC, Hsieh PH, et al. Potential clinical role of 18F FDG-PET/CT in detecting hip prosthesis infection: a study in patients undergoing two-stage revision arthroplasty with an interim spacer. Q J Nucl Med Mol Imaging 2010;54(4):429–35.

50. Kobayashi N, Inaba Y, Choe H, et al. Use of F-18 Fluoride PET to differentiate septic from aseptic loosening in total hip arthroplasty patients. Clin Nucl Med 2011;36(11):e156–61.

51. Choe H, Inaba Y, Kobayashi N, et al. Use of 18F-fluoride PET to determine the appropriate tissue sampling region for improved sensitivity of tissue examinations in cases of suspected periprosthetic infection after total hip arthroplasty. Acta Orthop 2011;82(4):427–32.

52. Zamora J, Abraira V, Muriel A, et al. Meta-DiSc: a software for meta-analysis of test accuracy data. BMC Med Res Methodol 2006;6:31.

FDG PET and PET/CT Imaging in Complicated Diabetic Foot

Sandip Basu, MBBS (Hons), DRM, DNB, MNAMS[a],
Hongming Zhuang, MD, PhD[b],
Abass Alavi, MD, PhD (Hon), DSc (Hon)[c],*

KEYWORDS

- FDG-PET • PET-CT • Diabetic foot

The pathogenesis of diabetic foot involves a multi-factorial mechanism and a complex pathophysiology (**Fig. 1**). The 2 primary factors are:

1. Diabetic neuropathy, which involves motor, sensory, and autonomic fibers.
2. Peripheral vascular disease, which involves the large vessels, and microvascular and capillary circulation.

The aforementioned 2 factors lead to (1) loss of protective sensation (owing to sensory neurodeficit) and (2) development of anatomic deformities (motor deficit). Both make the foot susceptible to repetitive trauma and ulceration. Superadded infection further complicates the situation and is difficult to manage owing to limited access of phagocytic cells and antibiotics because of impaired circulation related to peripheral vascular disease.

Another important entity is neuro-osteoarthropathy or Charcot arthropathy, where noninfectious soft tissue inflammation is associated with rapidly progressive destruction of joints and bone. Although osteomyelitis can be superimposed on Charcot arthropathy, this usually occurs in a well-vascularized and severely neuropathic foot that is nonulcerated. The pathogenesis typically involves minor trauma leading to fracture of a weakened bone and increase in the load on adjacent bone, leading to gross bone and joint destruction and persistent deformity. The persistent deformity increases the risk of secondary foot ulceration.

The estimated risk of a diabetic patient developing a foot ulcer in his or her lifetime has been proposed to be as high as 25%, and the annual incidence of foot ulcers has been estimated to be up to 2%.[1,2] In up to one-third of diabetic foot infections, osteomyelitis can supervene and is frequently the result of direct extension of the adjacent soft tissue infection, and represents a clinical challenge. This figure approximates 15% of the overall diabetic patients.[3]

POTENTIAL CLINICAL ROLE OF FDG-PET IN DIABETIC FOOT CARE

There are 3 settings in which [18-F] fluorodeoxyglucose (FDG)-PET or PET–computed tomography (CT)/PET–magnetic resonance (MR) imaging can have an important role in clinical decision making and will be most helpful to podiatrists if found accurate:

1. Diagnosis of deep soft tissue infection and osteomyelitis

[a] Radiation Medicine Centre, Bhabha Atomic Research Centre, Tata Memorial Hospital Annexe, Parel, Bombay 400012, India
[b] Division of Nuclear Medicine, Department of Radiology, The Children's Hospital of Philadelphia, University of Pennsylvania School of Medicine, 34th Street and Civic Center Boulevard, Philadelphia, PA 19104, USA
[c] Division of Nuclear Medicine, Department of Radiology, Hospital of the University of Pennsylvania, 3400 Spruce Street, Philadelphia, PA 19104, USA
* Corresponding author.
E-mail address: abass.alavi@uphs.upenn.edu

PET Clin 7 (2012) 151–160
doi:10.1016/j.cpet.2012.01.003
1556-8598/12/$ – see front matter © 2012 Published by Elsevier Inc

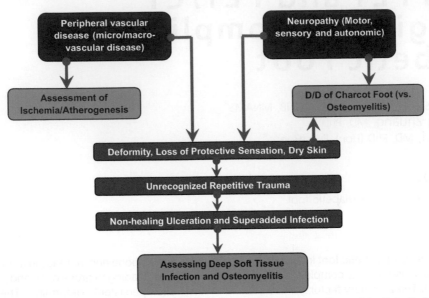

Fig. 1. Primary pathogenetic factors (*blue*), the further complicating factors (*brown*) in diabetic foot syndrome and diagnostic challenges where PET-CT/PET–MR imaging has a potential role (*green*). D/D, differential diagnosis.

2. Differentiating Charcot arthropathy from osteomyelitis
3. Evaluating the ischemia/atherogenesis component in a particular case.

Diagnosis of Deep Soft Tissue Infection and Osteomyelitis

Early diagnosis of osteomyelitis is important because antibiotic therapy can be curative and may prevent further complications, including amputation. The reported sensitivity and specificity of MR imaging is superior to plain radiography and CT and hence is considered the modality of choice for the evaluation of complicated diabetic foot, including osteomyelitis and other associated soft tissue abnormalities.

In a meta-analysis undertaken by Dinh and colleagues,[4] the pooled sensitivity and specificity, the summary measure of accuracy, and the diagnostic odds ratio were calculated with regard to accurate diagnosis of osteomyelitis underlying diabetic foot ulcers. The sensitivity and specificity of various methods were as follows: (1) exposed bone or probe-to-bone test 0.60 and 0.91; (2) plain film radiography (PFR) 0.54 and 0.68; (3) MR imaging 0.90 and 0.79; (4) bone scan 0.81 and 0.28; and (5) leukocyte scan 0.74 and 0.68. The diagnostic odds ratios for clinical examination, radiography, MR imaging, bone scan, and leukocyte scan were 49.45, 2.84, 24.36, 2.10, and 10.07, respectively. The investigators concluded the presence of exposed bone or a positive

probe-to-bone test result is moderately predictive of osteomyelitis and MR imaging is the most accurate imaging test for diagnosis of osteomyelitis.

FDG-PET and PET-CT imaging, thus, have been investigated for their potential in localizing deep infections of bone and soft tissue associated with the complicated diabetic foot. The combined PET-CT and PET–MR imaging fusion approaches offer unique tools for the diagnosis and management of the diabetic foot, which, through the establishment of appropriate diagnostic criteria, could emerge as highly accurate in this setting (**Figs. 2–7**).

Differentiating Charcot Arthropathy from Osteomyelitis

An important issue in the setting of diabetic foot syndrome is distinguishing osteomyelitis and neuro-osteoarthropathy (Charcot arthropathy). The usual clinical presentation of Charcot foot is a hot, swollen foot after minor trauma. Differentiating this from osteomyelitis, which can have a similar presentation, is a clinical challenge and is important, as the therapeutic approaches for these 2 limb-threatening complications are very different. The former is a self-limiting disease that is traditionally managed by immobilizing the foot in a cast and realignment arthrodesis of the hind foot, unless there is associated secondary ulceration and infection. The FDG uptake pattern, if different, can be useful in this area (see **Fig. 5**).

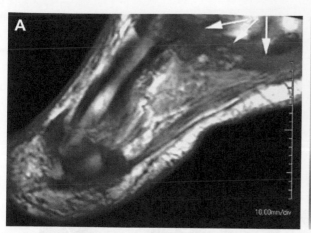
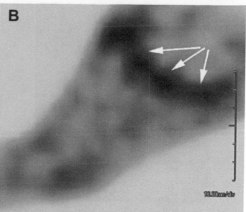

Fig. 2. Sixty-year-old woman with diabetes with suspected osteomyelitis. (*A*) MR image shows a linear area of abnormality at the junction of the tarsal metatarsal joint of the right foot (*arrows*) suggestive of osteomyelitis. (*B*) Corresponding to the same site, intense uptake of FDG is seen on PET image (*arrows*), which is also highly suggestive of infection. (*From* Nawaz A, Torigian DA, Siegelman ES, et al. Diagnostic performance of FDG-PET, MR imaging, and plain film radiography (PFR) for the diagnosis of osteomyelitis in the diabetic foot. Mol Imaging Biol 2010;12:335–42; with permission.)

Evaluating the Ischemia/Atherogenesis Component in a Particular Case

Peripheral vascular disease and peripheral neuropathy are postulated to play varying roles in the development of diabetic foot. The prevalence of these factors in patients is estimated to be as high as 40%, although no prospective study clearly documented their relative contribution. In a study aimed at estimating the relative contributions of neurologic and vascular abnormalities to the overall risk of diabetic foot ulceration, both neuropathy and vasculopathy were found to be strong independent risk factors for the development of diabetic foot ulcers. In this study, neuropathy was determined by vibratory, monofilament, and tendon reflex testing, whereas macrovascular disease was measured by ankle-arm blood pressure index and cutaneous perfusion was measured by transcutaneous oxygen tension on the dorsal foot.[5]

FDG-PET, by its ability to assess atherosclerosis in the large vessels of the lower limb, could help

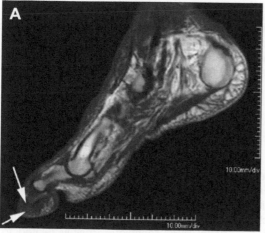
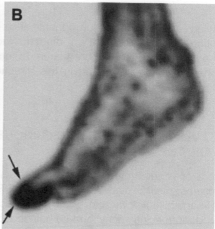

Fig. 3. Forty-one-year-old man with diabetes with history of long-standing chronic osteomyelitis of the left fourth metatarsal, neuropathic ulcer of the plantar surface of the left foot, and amputation of the left distal fifth digit. (*A*) T1-weighted sagittal MR image of the left foot demonstrate loss of signal intensity in the great toe region suggestive of osteomyelitis (*white arrow*). (*B*) PET image shows a focus of increased FDG uptake at the distal fourth metatarsal site (*black arrow*) corresponding to the abnormality noted on MR imaging. (*From* Nawaz A, Torigian DA, Siegelman ES, et al. Diagnostic performance of FDG-PET, MRI, and plain film radiography (PFR) for the diagnosis of osteomyelitis in the diabetic foot. Mol Imaging Biol 2010;12:335–42; with permission.)

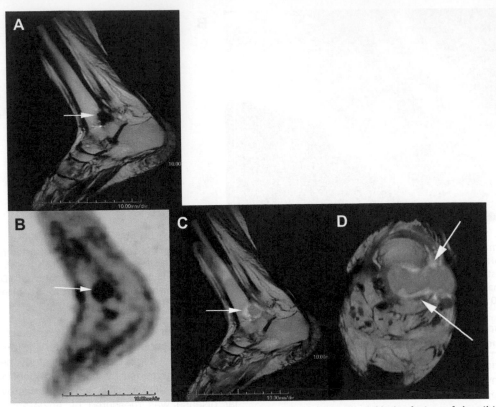

Fig. 4. 70-year-old woman with diabetes with history of resection of the distal fibula, fusion of the tibia-talar joint, and placement of orthopedic hardware. (*A*) MR image demonstrated chronic sinus tract extending from the lateral skin margin into the lateral distal tibia likely from prior hardware placement (*arrow*). The findings did not suggest osteomyelitis. (*B–D*) PET image demonstrates an abnormally increased focus of FDG uptake at the site (*arrows*), consistent with an active osteomyelitis. (*From* Nawaz A, Torigian DA, Siegelman ES, et al. Diagnostic performance of FDG-PET, MRI, and plain film radiography (PFR) for the diagnosis of osteomyelitis in the diabetic foot. Mol Imaging Biol 2010;12:335–42; with permission.)

in studying the ischemia component and its contribution the development of diabetic foot. This is a relatively less explored area to date and further research is required in this direction (**Figs. 8** and **9**).

FDG-PET VERSUS THE EXISTING TECHNIQUES: WHAT ARE THE ADVANTAGES?

A plethora of imaging modalities have been used for the management of diabetic foot, including PFR, CT, MR imaging, leukocyte scintigraphy, bone scintigraphy, gallium scintigraphy, and combined techniques. Of these, the 2 most important techniques have been MR imaging and leukocyte scintigraphy. Hence, the published studies with FDG-PET and PET-CT have been primarily aimed at validating and establishing the appropriate PET criteria for making a diagnosis of osteomyelitis and determining the accuracy of the technique through comparison with MR imaging and the labeled white blood cell (WBC) method.

The diagnosis of chronic osteomyelitis with anatomic imaging (eg, conventional radiography/CT/MR imaging) may prove difficult owing to the preexisting changes in the osseous architecture from prior trauma or surgery. In addition, FDG-PET is advantageous in the presence of metallic hardware. Despite the reported superiority over the other modalities, MR imaging demonstrates significant limitations for the diagnosis of osteomyelitis in the tarsal bones, hind foot, and in those with Charcot joints.[6–8]

There are several disadvantages of the conventional WBC technique, mainly related to procedures associated with the technical complexity of the labeled WBC method, coupled with the time required to complete the study. In addition, most infections associated with diabetic foot are subacute or chronic and hence the dominant inflammatory cells involved are monocytes and

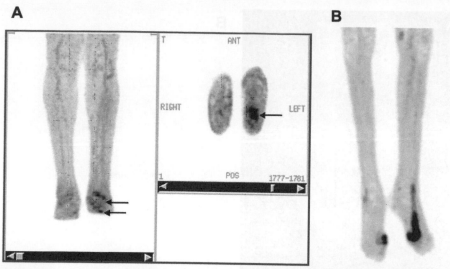

Fig. 5. (*A*) FDG-PET in a patient with diabetes mellitus demonstrating focal uptake in the ulcer (*arrows*) in the trans-axial images and the relatively low-grade diffuse uptake in the neuropathic osteoarthropathy (*arrows*) are clearly distinguishable from the uptake observed on the unaffected contralateral limb by visual inspection. (*B*) High-grade FDG uptake clearly distinctive from that of Charcot's neuroarthropathy. (*From* Basu S, Chryssikos T, Houseni M, et al. Potential role of FDG-PET in the setting of diabetic neuro-osteoarthropathy: can it differentiate uncomplicated Charcot's neuropathy from osteomyelitis and soft tissue infection? Nucl Med Commun 2007;28:465–72; with permission.)

lymphocytes. The labeled leukocyte preparation, on the other hand, primarily consists of neutrophils, which are predominantly observed in acute infections with neutrophilic infiltrate. Thus, labeled leukocytes are unlikely to detect chronic infection because very few monocytes and lymphocytes are labeled in such preparation. Prior therapy with antibiotics can further reduce the chemotropic effect of bacteria and, therefore, fewer leukocytes will migrate to the infectious sites. Both of these factors could make the labeled leukocyte method relatively less efficacious in this setting.

FDG-PET, in contrast, reflects "in vivo labeling" of the inflammatory cells residing at the site of infection and hence theoretically proposed to allow imaging a substantially larger population of cells.

In recent studies, PET scans have proved to demonstrate better accuracy in correctly diagnosing osteomyelitis compared with other modalities. In a meta-analysis, Termaat and colleagues[9] compared the efficacy of different imaging modalities in diagnosing chronic osteomyelitis. The investigators concluded that FDG-PET had the highest accuracy in confirming or excluding the

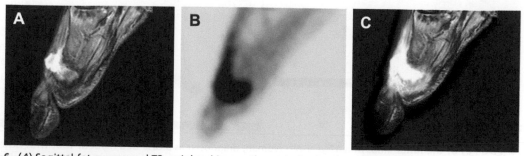

Fig. 6. (*A*) Sagittal fat-suppressed T2-weighted image through the forefoot demonstrates increased signal intensity within the distal metatarsal with osseous destruction and associated fluid in adjacent soft tissue, in keeping with osteomyelitis. (*B*) Sagittal FDG-PET image through the corresponding location demonstrates increased FDG-uptake in the corresponding location, consistent with osteomyelitis. (*C*) Coregistered FDG-PET and MR image of a patient with diabetic foot and suspected bone infection in the distal metatarsal. (*From* Nawaz A, Torigian DA, Siegelman ES, et al. Diagnostic performance of FDG-PET, MRI, and plain film radiography (PFR) for the diagnosis of osteomyelitis in the diabetic foot. Mol Imaging Biol 2010;12:335–42; with permission.)

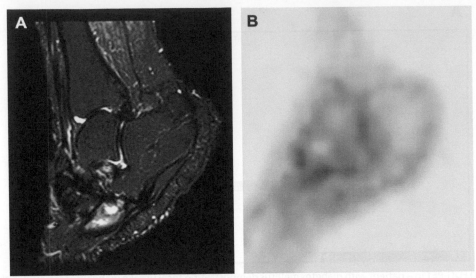

Fig. 7. (*A*) Sagittal fat-suppressed T2-weighted image through the hindfoot/ankle demonstrates trace fluid in the talocalcaneal joint space. No gross osseous destruction or erosions are seen. (*B*) Sagittal FDG-PET image through the corresponding location demonstrates mild FDG-uptake in the location of the talocalcaneal joint, indicative of Charcot arthropathy. Surgical pathology result suggested no infection. (*From* Nawaz A, Torigian DA, Siegelman ES, et al. Diagnostic performance of FDG-PET, MRI, and plain film radiography (PFR) for the diagnosis of osteomyelitis in the diabetic foot. Mol Imaging Biol 2010;12:335–42; with permission.)

diagnosis of chronic osteomyelitis with a pooled sensitivity of 96% and a pooled specificity of 91%.

ANALYSIS OF PUBLISHED DATA ON USING FDG-PET IN THE DIABETIC FOOT

The literature on the efficacy of FDG-PET in reliably diagnosing or excluding osteomyelitis in the diabetic foot is divided and clearly there appear to be 2 groups of results: one emphasizing the potential usefulness and the other depicting a low sensitivity of this modality (**Table 1**). The latter (ie, those reporting limited utility), as one can observe, has been examined in fewer patients. PET-CT was used in 2 studies ,whereas 4 studies reported efficacy with FDG-PET alone. The

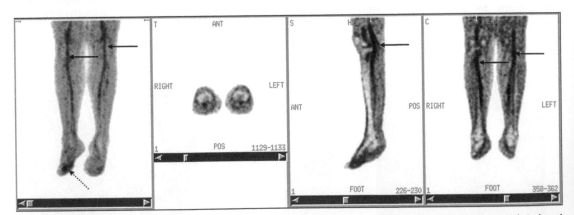

Fig. 8. FDG-PET of the lower limbs of a 47-year-old woman, diagnosed as a case of a diabetic foot with ischemic complications. FDG-PET demonstrated prominent diffuse uptake in the lower extremity arteries (*arrows*) including popliteal and tibial arteries. In addition to showing diffuse FDG uptake in the arteries, focal intense FDG uptake was noted in the right great toe corresponding to the clinical evidence of a gangrenous right toe (FDG uptake marked by *broken arrow*). Although low-grade FDG uptake is observed at times in normal limbs, the FDG uptake in the popliteal and tibial arteries in the present case was high grade and quite distinctive from those of normal extremities. (*From* Basu S, Zhuang H, Alavi A. Imaging of lower extremity artery atherosclerosis in diabetic foot: FDG-PET imaging and histopathological correlates. Clin Nucl Med 2007;32(7):567–8; with permission.)

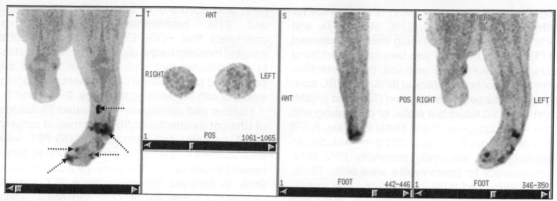

Fig. 9. FDG-PET of lower extremities of a 60-year-old woman, diagnosed as a case of neuropathic Charcot foot. Increased FDG uptake was noted in the distal left tibia just above the ankle, midshaft of the tibia, and in the soft tissue of the lateral and plantar aspects of the left foot, which was suggestive of osteomyelitis and cellulitis respectively (*broken arrows*), consequent to the neuropathy. No uptake was observed in the arteries. Histopathological correlation was available in both cases shown in Figs. 8 and 9: the case showing diffuse FDG uptake in the arteries (see **Fig. 8**) revealed features of atherosclerosis along with evidence of a gangrenous right toe; the other case without any uptake in the arteries (Fig. 9) had no evidence of atherosclerosis on pathologic examination. (*From* Basu S, Zhuang H, Alavi A. Imaging of lower extremity artery atherosclerosis in diabetic foot: FDG-PET imaging and histopathological correlates. Clin Nucl Med 2007;32(7):567–8; with permission.)

comparably low spatial resolution, a frequently cited shortcoming of FDG-PET alone, can be overcome with the combined modality FDG-PET/CT, which allows better anatomic localization that is crucial for accurately diagnosing osteomyelitis from that of adjacent soft tissue infection.

In a prospective study, Schwegler and colleagues[10] evaluated 20 diabetic patients with a chronic foot ulcer (>8 weeks) without antibiotic pretreatment and without clinical signs for osteomyelitis and compared the value of MR imaging, FDG-PET, and 99mTc-labeled monoclonal antigranulocyte antibody scintigraphy (99mTc-MOAB). Histopathological confirmation of the final diagnosis was available for 7 patients with suggestive scans. In this limited cohort, MR imaging was positive in 6 of the 7 patients with proven osteomyelitis, whereas 18F-FDG-PET and 99mTc-MOAB

were positive only in (the same) 2 patients. The investigators recommended MR imaging as the imaging modality of choice in diagnosing or excluding osteomyelitis in the diabetic foot.

In another study,[11] the value of sequential FDG-PET/CT was prospectively examined in patients with a high suspicion of osteomyelitis to define the objective interpretation criteria and the result was compared with WBC scintigraphy. A total of 13 patients were enrolled and a biopsy or tissue culture was performed for final diagnosis. In this study, the following criteria were used to diagnose infection: a maximal standardized uptake value (SUVmax) greater than 2.0 after 1 and 2 hours but stable or decreasing with time was suggestive of a soft tissue infection. An SUVmax less than 2.0 excluded an infection. Using these criteria, sensitivity, specificity, positive predictive value (PPV),

Table 1
Reported studies examining the role of FDG-PET/PET-CT in diabetic foot syndrome

Study (First Author, Year)	No. Patients	Charcot Arthropathy Separately Analyzed	PET Alone/PET-CT	Conclusion (Useful/Limited Accuracy)
Hopfner et al,[14] 2004	16	Yes	PET alone	Useful
Keidar et al,[12] 2005	18	No	PET-CT	Useful
Basu et al,[15] 2007	63	Yes	PET alone	Useful
Schwegler et al,[10] 2008	20	No	PET alone	Limited accuracy
Nawaz et al,[13] 2010	110	No	PET alone	Useful
Familiari et al,[11] 2011	13	No	PET-CT	Limited accuracy

Abbreviation: CT, computed tomography.

negative predictive value (NPV), and accuracy for osteomyelitis were 43%, 67%, 60%, 50%, and 54%, respectively. Combining visual assessment of PET at 1 hour and CT was best for differentiating between osteomyelitis and soft tissue infection, with a diagnostic accuracy of 62%. For WBC scintigraphy, a target to background (T/B) ratio greater than 2.0 at 20 hours but stable or decreasing with time was suggestive of soft tissue infection. A T/B ratio of no more than 2.0 at 20 hours excluded an infection. Thus, sensitivity, specificity, PPV, NPV, and accuracy for osteomyelitis were 86%, 100%, 100%, 86%, and 92%, respectively. The investigators concluded that FDG-PET/CT, even with sequential imaging, has a low diagnostic accuracy for osteomyelitis and cannot replace WBC scintigraphy in patients with diabetic foot.

In one of the earliest reports with PET-CT, Keidar and colleagues[12] evaluated 14 diabetic patients with 18 clinically suspected sites of infection; PET, CT, and hybrid images were independently evaluated for the diagnosis and localization of an infectious process. Open wounds or ulcers were present in 12 of the 18 sites. PET/CT correctly localized 8 foci in 4 patients to bone, indicating osteomyelitis, whereas it correctly excluded osteomyelitis in 5 foci in 5 patients, with the abnormal 18F-FDG uptake limited to infected soft tissues only. The accuracy of ^{18}F-FDG-PET/CT in this investigation was about 94%. The mean SUVmax in infectious foci was 5.7 (range, 1.7–11.1) for both osseous and soft tissue sites of infection. The investigators found no relationship between the patients' glycemic state and the degree of ^{18}F-FDG uptake. They recommended FDG-PET for the diagnosis of diabetes-related infection and concluded that precise anatomic localization of increased 18F-FDG uptake provided by PET/CT enables accurate differentiation between osteomyelitis and soft tissue infection.

Nawaz and colleagues[13] reported the analyzed results from 110 prospectively investigated diabetic patients at the hospital of the University of Pennsylvania, where a head-to-head comparison was made between FDG-PET, MR imaging, and PFR of the feet. They obtained promising results with FDG-PET, which correctly diagnosed osteomyelitis in 21 of 26 patients and correctly excluded it in 74 of 80, with sensitivity, specificity, PPV, NPV, and accuracy of 81%, 93%, 78%, 94%, and 90%, respectively. MR imaging correctly diagnosed osteomyelitis in 20 of 22 and correctly excluded it in 56 of 72, with sensitivity, specificity, PPV, NPV, and accuracy of 91%, 70%, 56%, 97%, and 81%, respectively. PFR correctly diagnosed osteomyelitis in 15 of 24 and correctly excluded it in 65 of 75, with sensitivity, specificity, PPV,

NPV, and accuracy of 63%, 87%, 60%, 88%, and 81%, respectively. The investigators concluded that FDG-PET is a highly specific imaging modality for the diagnosis of osteomyelitis in the diabetic foot and, therefore, should be considered to be a useful complementary imaging modality with MR imaging (see **Figs. 2–4, 6**, and **7**).

Hopfner and colleagues[14] evaluated 39 lesions of Charcot osteoarthropathy confirmed at surgery in 16 patients, and noted that FDG-PET with a dedicated full-ring PET scanner accurately diagnosed this disorder in 37 lesions, for a sensitivity of 95%. In contrast, the coincidence PET camera provided a sensitivity of 77% and MR imaging had a sensitivity of 79%. The mean SUVmax in the Charcot arthropathy lesions was 1.8 (range, 0.5–4.1). Those investigators concluded that FDG-PET can correctly distinguish osteomyelitis from Charcot osteoarthropathy and may be preferable to radiography and MR imaging in the preoperative evaluation of patients with Charcot neuroarthropathy of the foot.

Another analysis from a prospective research study by Basu and colleagues[15] also demonstrated promising results in diagnosing osteomyelitis and differentiating it from Charcot foot. In this study, a total of 63 patients in 4 groups were evaluated. A low degree of diffuse FDG uptake that was clearly distinguishable from that of normal joints was observed in joints of patients with Charcot osteoarthropathy. The SUVmax in lesions of patients with Charcot osteoarthropathy varied from 0.7 to 2.4 (mean, 1.3 ± 0.4), whereas those of the midfoot of the healthy control subjects and the uncomplicated diabetic foot ranged from 0.2 to 0.7 (mean, 0.42 ± 0.12) and from 0.2 to 0.8 (mean, 0.5 ± 0.16), respectively. The only patient with Charcot osteoarthropathy with superimposed osteomyelitis in this series had an SUVmax of 6.5. The SUVmax of the sites of osteomyelitis as a complication of diabetic foot was 2.9 to 6.2 (mean, 4.38 ± 0.39). An unifactorial analysis of variance test yielded a statistical significance in the SUVmax among the 4 groups (P<.01). The SUVmax value differences between the healthy control groups and the uncomplicated diabetic foot were not statistically significant by the Student t test (P>.05). The overall sensitivity and accuracy of FDG-PET in the diagnosis of Charcot osteoarthropathy were 100.0% and 93.8%, respectively, and those for MR imaging were 76.9% and 75.0%, respectively. The investigators concluded that these results underscored the valuable role of FDG-PET in the setting of Charcot neuroarthropathy by reliably differentiating it from osteomyelitis, both in general and when foot ulcer is present (see **Fig. 5**).

In a recent commentary,[16] the discordance of results has been proposed to be attributable to the heterogeneity of the study population, such as type of diabetes, temporal relation between administration of insulin or oral agents and injection of FDG, presence or absence of vascular insufficiency, reference standard used in the studies for comparison, and so on. Further studies may clarify these points.

Assessment of Arterial Insufficiency in a Particular Case

As mentioned previously, with regard to assessing the ischemia component and its contribution in the development of the diabetic foot, FDG-PET could help by its ability to image atherosclerosis in the large vessels of the lower limb. Relatively little research[17,18] has been done in this area and it is expected that further research will address this topic (see **Figs. 8** and **9**).

SUMMARY

It is expected that with further published research, the role and reliability of PET-CT and PET–MR imaging in diabetic foot syndrome will be clearly defined. Certainly, the combined PET-CT fusion approach appears better than FDG-PET imaging alone, owing to better anatomic localization and thereby aiding in differentiation of soft tissue infection and bone more precisely.[19,20] We believe PET–MR imaging may emerge as the diagnostic procedure of choice in the management of these patients and will be able to address the most challenging questions associated with the complications.

ACKNOWLEDGMENTS

The authors thank B. Basu for helping in preparing the schematic diagram of **Fig. 1**.

REFERENCES

1. Abbott CA, Carrington AL, Ashe H, et al. The North-West Diabetes Foot Care Study: incidence of, and risk factors for, new diabetic foot ulceration in a community-based patient cohort. Diabet Med 2002;19:377–84.
2. Reiber GE, Vileikyte L, Boyko EJ, et al. Causal pathways for incident lower-extremity ulcers in patients with diabetes from two settings. Diabetes Care 1999;22:157–62.
3. Marcus CD, Ladam-Marcus VJ, Leone J, et al. MR imaging of osteomyelitis and neuropathic osteoarthropathy in the feet of diabetics. Radiographics 1996; 16:1337–48.
4. Dinh MT, Abad CL, Safdar N. Diagnostic accuracy of physical examination and imaging tests for osteomyelitis underlying diabetic foot ulcers: meta analysis. Clin Infect Dis 2008;47(4):519–27.
5. McNeely MJ, Boyko EJ, Ahroni JH, et al. The independent contributions of diabetic neuropathy and vasculopathy in foot ulceration. How great are the risks? Diabetes Care 1995;18(2):216–9.
6. Craig JG, Amin MB, Wu K, et al. Osteomyelitis of the diabetic foot: MR imaging-pathologic correlation. Radiology 1997;203:849–55.
7. Lipman BT, Collier BD, Carrera GF, et al. Detection of osteomyelitis in the neuropathic foot: nuclear medicine, MRI and conventional radiography. Clin Nucl Med 1998;23:77–82.
8. Yansouni CP, Mak A, Libman MD. Limitations of magnetic resonance imaging in the diagnosis of osteomyelitis underlying diabetic foot ulcers. Clin Infect Dis 2009;48(1):135.
9. Termaat MF, Rajimakers PG, Scholten HJ, et al. The accuracy of diagnostic imaging for the assessment of chronic osteomyelitis: a systematic review and meta analysis. J Bone Joint Surg Am 2005;87(11): 2464–71.
10. Schwegler B, Stumpe KD, Weishaupt D, et al. Unsuspected osteomyelitis is frequent in persistent diabetic foot ulcer and better diagnosed by MRI than by 18F-FDG PET or 99mTc-MOAB. J Intern Med 2008;263:99–106.
11. Familiari D, Glaudemans AW, Vitale V, et al. Can sequential 18F-FDG-PET/CT replace WBC imaging in the diabetic foot? J Nucl Med 2011;52:1012–9.
12. Keidar Z, Militianu D, Melamed E, et al. The diabetic foot: initial experience with 18F-FDG-PET/CT. J Nucl Med 2005;46:444–9.
13. Nawaz A, Torigian DA, Siegelman ES, et al. Diagnostic performance of FDG-PET, MRI, and plain film radiography (PFR) for the diagnosis of osteomyelitis in the diabetic foot. Mol Imaging Biol 2010;12: 335–42.
14. Hopfner S, Krolak C, Kessler S, et al. Preoperative imaging of Charcot neuroarthropathy in diabetic patients: comparison of ring PET, hybrid PET, and magnetic resonance imaging. Foot Ankle Int 2004; 25:890–5.
15. Basu S, Chryssikos T, Houseni M, et al. Potential role of FDG-PET in the setting of diabetic neuro-osteoarthropathy: can it differentiate uncomplicated Charcot's neuropathy from osteomyelitis and soft tissue infection? Nucl Med Commun 2007;28:465–72.
16. Palestro CJ. 18F-FDG and diabetic foot infections: the verdict is. J Nucl Med 2011;52(7):1009–11.
17. Basu S, Zhuang H, Alavi A. Imaging of lower extremity artery atherosclerosis in diabetic foot: FDG-PET imaging and histopathological correlates. Clin Nucl Med 2007;32(7):567–8.

18. Basu S, Shah J, Houseni M, et al. Uptake in the lower extremity arteries in diabetic foot with ischemic complications and neuropathic osteoarthropathy: FDG PET and Histopathological correlation. Clin Nucl Med 2008;33(1):74–80 [Abstracts from the ACNP 34th Annual Meeting. February 15–18, San Antonio, TX, 2007.].

19. Basu S, Chryssikos T, Moghadam-Kia S, et al. Positron emission tomography as a diagnostic tool in infection: present role and future possibilities. Semin Nucl Med 2009;39(1):36–51.

20. Basu S, Zhuang H, Torigian DA, et al. Functional imaging of inflammatory diseases using nuclear medicine techniques. Semin Nucl Med 2009;39(2):124–45.

FDG PET Assessment of Osteomyelitis: A Review

Phyllis Dioguardi, MD, MA[a],*, Santosh R. Gaddam, MD[a],
Hongming Zhuang, MD, PhD[b], Drew A. Torigian, MD, MA[c],
Abass Alavi, MD, PhD (Hon), DSc (Hon)[a]

KEYWORDS

- FDG-PET • PET/CT • Osteomyelitis
- Musculoskeletal infection • Radionuclide imaging
- Chronic osteomyelitis • Prosthesis-related infections
- Complicated diabetic foot

The ability to identify infection quickly and accurately is a major goal of diagnostic medicine because, despite greater understanding of how infection is caused and how it evolves, it remains a major source of patient morbidity and mortality worldwide. Early diagnosis and exclusion of infection and inflammation are of the utmost importance for optimal management of patients with infections such as osteomyelitis. Despite important advances in surgical and long-term antibiotic treatment, it often remains refractory to therapy, leading to chronic illness. The diagnosis of chronic infection may be difficult, because signs and symptoms may be absent. Because the infection often develops in an indirect manner and threatens to relapse, the diagnosis of posttraumatic/postsurgical osteomyelitis is usually made from a combination of clinical, laboratory, and imaging examinations. Together with the involved clinician, surgeon, microbiologist, and pathologist, the radiologist and nuclear medicine physician have to make use of all available information to exclude or confirm the presence of active infection or further complications of the disease.[1]

Imaging plays an increasing role in the care of patients with infectious and inflammatory diseases.

Structural imaging such as plain film radiography, computed tomography (CT), and magnetic resonance (MR) imaging is most commonly used to detect and localize structural changes that have developed because of infection and inflammation. More recently, functional and molecular imaging methods have been developed (eg, [^{18}F]fluorodeoxyglucose [FDG] PET) that are complementary to structural imaging modalities and are proving effective in guiding the care of patients with infectious and inflammatory disorders. Nuclear medicine has for a long time focused its attention on the use of molecular imaging to enhance the rapid and accurate identification and localization of infections (particularly osteomyelitis) that may occur following trauma, in association with joint prosthesis, or in the feet of patients with diabetes mellitus. Several molecular imaging agents are already in clinical use, including labeled antibacterial agents, labeled antimicrobial peptides, monoclonal antibodies for leukocyte labeling, and labeled liposomes. Foremost among these imaging agents is FDG, which has been touted as the molecule of the millennium.

FDG-PET has an established record of efficacy in the assessment and detection of a variety of

[a] Division of Nuclear Medicine, Department of Radiology, Hospital of the University of Pennsylvania, 3400 Spruce Street, Philadelphia, PA 19104, USA
[b] Division of Nuclear Medicine, Department of Radiology, The Children's Hospital of Philadelphia, University of Pennsylvania School of Medicine, 34th Street and Civic Center Boulevard, Philadelphia, PA 19104, USA
[c] Department of Radiology, Hospital of the University of Pennsylvania, 3400 Spruce Street, Philadelphia, PA 19104, USA
* Corresponding author.
E-mail address: phyllis.dioguardi@uphs.upenn.edu

PET Clin 7 (2012) 161–179
doi:10.1016/j.cpet.2012.01.011
1556-8598/12/$ – see front matter © 2012 Published by Elsevier Inc

nononcologic disease conditions. The diagnosis of infection and the ability to distinguish bacterial infection from nonbacterial inflammation through the use of PET has gained interest in recent years. With modern advances, FDG-PET is becoming a more widely accepted modality for identifying a diverse group of infectious and inflammatory processes, such as osteomyelitis, prosthesis-related infections, spondylodiscitis, sarcoidosis, and infections related to acquired immunodeficiency syndrome(AIDS), and is useful for the evaluation of patients with fever of unknown origin (FUO). However, FDG and other radionuclide imaging agents target components of these inflammatory responses, none of which are infection specific. In spite of the success of FDG-PET in oncology, the test is not specific for malignancy. FDG-PET is a method to identify cells and tissues with an increased metabolic (glycolytic) rate. Because accelerated energy metabolism is not specific to cancer, many noncancerous tissues take up FDG, and false-positive findings are common. Consequently, This article provides a survey of the most important current applications of FDG-PET in osteomyelitis and notes the specific technical and/or diagnostic challenges in any given application.[2]

RADIOTRACERS

Radiotracers for the detection and localization of infectious and inflammatory processes have been used since the 1950s. The radiotracers used to diagnose bone infection are divided into 2 groups: the first group comprises infection/inflammation seeking agents, which include ^{67}Ga, radiolabeled antigranulocyte antibodies, and radiolabeled leukocytes for white blood cell (WBC) scintigraphy; the second group contains agents that reflect metabolic changes associated with infection/inflammation, such as radiolabeled diphosphonates for bone scintigraphy. The introduction of radiotracers in nuclear medicine has enhanced infection imaging, because they depend on the demonstration of pathophysiologic changes, which occur earlier in the infectious process and also resolve quickly after cure of the infection compared with gross anatomic changes in osseous structure as detected by conventional imaging modalities. Ideally, radiotracers developed for the detection of infection and inflammation should be highly sensitive and able to distinguish between infectious and noninfectious inflammation. Recently, a wide variety of radiotracers have been tested for imaging infectious and inflammation processes in the hopes of achieving the desirable characteristic of high specificity. Currently, there are only a few agents in use for infection and inflammation imaging. These agents include FDG, autologous WBC labeled with ^{99m}Tc-hexamethylpropylene amine oxime or ^{111}In-oxine, ^{99m}Tc-labeled diphosphonates such as methylene diphosphonate (MDP) or hydroxymethylene diphosphonate, ^{67}Ga-citrate, ^{99m}Tc-labeled nanocolloids, and ^{99m}Tc-labeled or ^{111}In-labeled proteins, such as immunoglobulin (Ig) G or albumin. The main limitation of these techniques is lack of specificity, because these methods target/label components of the inflammatory response itself, such as immune globulin, neutrophils, and cytokines. Thus, these established methods are inflammation specific but do not adequately distinguish between infectious and noninfectious inflammation.[1,3]

Infection-specific imaging is performed with a variety of radiotracers that all label one of the consecutive steps of the host response to the invading organisms. Acute inflammation is characterized by hyperemia, increased endothelial permeability, exudation of proteins, and cellular migration predominantly involving granulocytes, whereas, in chronic infection, hyperemia and increased endothelial permeability are less prominent and infiltration with macrophages and lymphocytes is predominant. The choice of the optimal radiotracer therefore depends on the grade of inflammation, age of infection, availability, cost, and radiation exposure.[4]

The accumulation of these agents in inflamed tissue is based on different mechanisms. The first mechanism is uptake into inflamed tissue as a result of increased metabolism, either of inflammatory cells ([^{18}F]FDG, as a glucose analogue reflecting the energy demand of inflammatory cells) or of tissue-specific cells with increased activity as a reaction to inflammation (^{99m}Tc-MDP), reflecting the activity of osteoblasts as the active response of bone to inflammation. The second mechanism is nonspecific accumulation in the site of inflammation as a result of increased blood flow and enhanced vascular permeability (albumin, IgG). In the case of labeled activated leukocytes, the uptake mechanism involves intact chemotaxis and specific migration to the site of inflammation. ^{67}Ga-citrate binds to transferrin, with the complex undergoing extravasation at sites of inflammation because of increased blood flow and increased vascular permeability. ^{67}Ga-citrate also binds to lactoferrin, which is present in high concentrations in inflammatory foci. Most radiolabeled agents accumulate at sites of infection if the local blood flow and the vascular permeability are increased, but diphosphonates are unique in that several different mechanisms play a role in the accumulation of these radiotracers. Diphosphonates show increased uptake at sites of inflammation on early images taken directly after injection of the radiotracer (arterial phase, as a result of increased blood flow) and a few minutes after injection (blood pool phase, as a result of increased vascular permeability in combination with increased blood flow) and on the delayed images several hours after injection (static phase, as a result of increased bone metabolism reflecting osteoblastic activity at sites of inflammation).[4]

APPROACH

The approach to diagnosis of a specific inflammatory disease depends on the type of suspected disease and the clinical presentation. Therefore, the context in which imaging procedures are used varies considerably. For many inflammatory and infectious diseases, no definitive guidelines for the use of imaging procedures exist, but in some cases there is sufficient evidence from the literature to provide guidance for the use of particular imaging procedures for optimal diagnosis or follow-up of disease conditions of interest.

From a clinical point of view, imaging should provide all of the information needed to confirm or exclude the diagnosis of osteomyelitis. Following the decision between conservative or surgical therapy, additional information may be needed for planning subsequent procedures and treatment. Therefore, the value of imaging depends on the sensitivity and specificity of the various imaging modalities. From a clinical standpoint, imaging should strive to provide answers to the following questions concerning osteomyelitis:

1. Is this infection and noninfectious inflammation?
2. Is this acute or chronic infection?
3. Where is the main focus of infection? Are there other infectious foci, and where are their locations?
4. Which adjacent tissues or structures are involved, if any?
5. What is the local quality and vitality of bone and surrounding tissues?
6. Are there associated complications? Is there adequate assessment of prosthetic involvement?
7. Has there been a therapeutic response to treatment?

The value of conventional radionuclide imaging techniques commonly used to diagnose osteomyelitis depends on the sensitivity and specificity of the different imaging procedures. For example, 3-phase bone scintigraphy is sensitive for osteomyelitis. However, in the setting of bone with preexisting conditions, which include trauma, presence of prosthetic hardware, and neuropathic joint disease,

3-bone scintigraphy is less reliable for accurately distinguishing uncomplicated bone healing from osteomyelitis because of continuous bone turnover, which is present in both conditions. In the case of traumatized bone following fracture, it is common for increased ^{99m}Tc-MDP levels to persist for many years, making the diagnosis of posttraumatic osteomyelitis especially challenging. Persistent MDP uptake can also make evaluation of therapeutic treatment response difficult, because increased MDP activity may persist long after successful treatment has been completed. In these situations, dual radiotracer studies are often used: sequential bone gallium, combined bone leukocyte, or, in most cases, combined leukocyte–bone marrow imaging.[5] However, these dual radiotracer studies also have important limitations and drawbacks. For example, the need for additional imaging adds to the complexity and cost of these studies, as well as inconvenience to patients, many of whom are elderly and debilitated. Limitations are also noted with labeled leukocyte imaging, particularly the in vitro labeling process, which is labor intensive, often unavailable, and requires direct contact with blood products.

When used for suspected osteomyelitis, a 3-phase bone scan with ^{99m}Tc-labeled diphosphonates (MDP, hexose diphosphate, dicarboxypropandiphosphate, hydroxyethylidenedisphosphanate) has often been the standard method performed. Three-phase bone scintigraphy is the most widely used nuclear imaging procedure for the evaluation of osseous infections because of its availability and low cost.[6] Bone scintigraphy is extremely sensitive (exceeding 90%), but has a limited specificity, only up to 50%.[7] The limited specificity is explained by uptake of radiotracer at all sites of increased bone metabolism irrespective of the underlying cause. The low specificity of bone scintigraphy poses a challenge for accurate diagnosis of osteomyelitis, particularly when complicating conditions are superimposed, such as neuropathic osteoarthropathy, postsurgical changes, healing fractures, and chronic infections. However, if combined single-photon emission computed tomography (SPECT)/CT is performed, the specificity increases to more than 80%.[8] As an alternative to bone scanning, labeled leukocyte imaging has been proposed. However, because of physiologic uptake into bone marrow, both sensitivity and specificity may be impaired. Therefore, combined imaging with labeled leukocytes and sulfur colloids for bone marrow has been evaluated. Both labeled leukocytes and sulfur colloid accumulate in the bone marrow; leukocytes also accumulate in infection, whereas sulfur colloid does not. The combined study is positive for infection when activity is present on the labeled leukocyte image without corresponding activity on the sulfur colloid marrow image. This combined imaging approach results in increased sensitivity and specificity values, both of which are more than 90%.[9] In addition, the combination of WBC and bone marrow scans results in high sensitivities and specificities of more than 90%. This combination has been shown to be superior to MR imaging and CT in postoperative patients with osteomyelitis. However, for detection of vertebral osteomyelitis, WBC imaging has low sensitivity (~50%), which has been hypothesized to reflect the inability of leukocytes to migrate into the encapsulated infection or into areas that have a lower blood supply, particularly within the axial skeleton. The photopenic lesions or cold defects, which are not specific for infection, together with the physiologic uptake of WBCs into the bone marrow, hamper accurate detection of vertebral infection. In contrast, in peripheral bones, especially after orthopedic surgery, there is often displacement of bone marrow resulting in areas of increased uptake or hot spots that must be distinguished from focal infection.

In these situations, combined bone gallium, bone leukocyte, or leukocyte–bone marrow imaging can be used; however, specificities still vary between 50% and 100%.[10][111]In-labeled leukocyte imaging is frequently used to identify infectious foci in the peripheral skeleton.[11][111]In-labeled leukocyte scintigraphy combined with ^{99m}Tc-MDP scintigraphy is the imaging method of choice for posttraumatic infection imaging at fracture nonunion sites.[10] However, the frequent need to perform 2 examinations and to image at multiple times is not only inconvenient to patients but also adds to the overall radiation dose. Another concern is the blood handling process, including separating, labeling, and reinjecting WBCs, which may result in suboptimal preparation and may introduce infection.

Specificity for detecting and monitoring infectious processes by conventional planar scintigraphy can be improved by performing SPECT,[8,12] and by using other structural imaging techniques, including conventional radiography, CT, MR imaging, and ultrasonography (US). Some findings of acute osteomyelitis on CT include osteolysis of cortical bone, presence of small foci of gas, and increased enhancement after administration of contrast media. MR imaging has a high sensitivity for detection of osteomyelitis and soft tissue infection and provides high spatial and soft tissue contrast resolution for delineation of the spatial extent of osteomyelitis. MR imaging is particularly useful in detection of osteomyelitis and discitis involving the axial skeleton.[13] However, both CT and MR imaging lack specificity in chronic

infection and in the presence of prosthetic joint replacements because of associated susceptibility artifacts. In addition, these modalities are limited in their ability to detect and characterize acute or chronic infection in previously altered bone, such as in the setting of prior surgery or prior trauma.[14] The structural alterations of bone in chronic infection can persist intermittently for years. Even with intravenous administration of contrast media it is difficult to distinguish latent infection from bone remodeling by either CT or MR imaging. Anatomic changes often take some time to become visible, may not always be present, and their resolution may lag behind cure of the infection. However, one modality, FDG-PET, is capable of reliably and accurately confirming presence or absence of osteomyelitis in posttraumatic and postsurgical conditions.

MOLECULAR BASIS OF FDG-PET

FDG-PET/CT is commonly used for staging and therapy response assessment of malignant tumors. There is a long history of the use of FDG-PET in oncology for the staging and grading of tumors. The high rate of aerobic glycolysis in proliferating tumor cells is central in the increased uptake of FDG in malignant cells. FDG is transported into tumor cells through glucose transport proteins (GLUT) such as GLUT 1 and GLUT 3, which are typically upregulated in tumor cells. Once FDG is internalized, it is phosphorylated by hexokinase to FDG-6-phosphate. Unlike glucose-6-phosphate, FDG-6-phosphate does not enter glycolysis because of the presence of fluorine substitution at the 2 position, and thus becomes metabolically trapped. It is the subsequent accumulation of FDG in metabolically active cells that provides contrast on FDG-PET imaging.[15]

Much like tumor cells, inflammatory cells exhibit a hyperglycolytic state during infection.[16] The mechanism for FDG uptake in inflammatory cells is the overexpression of GLUT 1 and GLUT 3 in macrophages, neutrophils, and lymphocytes stimulated by various cytokines and growth factors. In activated inflammatory cells, there are not only an increased number and expression of these glucose transporters but also an increased affinity of these transporters for deoxyglucose.[17,18]

DIAGNOSTIC IMAGING ASSESSMENT OF CHRONIC OSTEOMYELITIS VERSUS REPARATIVE BONE HEALING

Healthy bone is resistant to bacterial colonization and infection; however, in the setting of traumatized bone, necrosis, foreign bodies, and predisposing factors including diabetes mellitus, chronic renal failure, immunodeficiency states, such as AIDS, chronic alcoholism, and drug addiction, bone becomes more vulnerable to infection. Trauma can have a detrimental effect because of the host response to infection through activation of cytokines. The resulting compromised microcirculation may lead to exacerbation of tissue necrosis in already devitalized and necrotic bone. These nonliving, necrotic surfaces, along with the presence of prostheses and local hematoma, provide an excellent culture medium for bacterial growth. As previously mentioned, the glycocalyx (biofilm) is a carbohydrate-enriched coating produced by bacteria that provides a protective coat from both host factors and antibiotics, enhancing the ability of bacteria to establish an infection.[19]

Osteomyelitis is often categorized as acute, subacute, or chronic, with the classification of each type based on the time of disease onset. Acute osteomyelitis develops within 2 weeks after disease onset, subacute osteomyelitis within 1 to several months, and chronic osteomyelitis after a few months. Weiland and colleagues[20] chose a period of 6 months to distinguish between acute and chronic osteomyelitis. Schauwecker[21] stated that osteomyelitis requiring more than 1 episode of treatment and/or a persistent infection lasting more than 6 weeks should be considered as chronic. Termaat and colleagues[22] also preferred the Schauwecker[21] classification because it provides a clear cutoff for acute and chronic osteomyelitis, emphasizing that the 6-week period is more than 3 times longer than the 10-day period during which bone necrosis occurs in acute osteomyelitis. Several formal classification systems for osteomyelitis based on the cause, the physiology of the host, or on soft tissue and osseous defects have also been published. The classification by Waldvogel and colleagues[23] is old, but still topical, and is based on the genesis of osteomyelitis (hematogenous or secondary) and on the modality of onset. Acute hematogenous osteomyelitis symptoms last no more than 10 days. The chronic form is the most frequent and includes all the remaining cases (**Table 1**). The classification by Cierny and colleagues[24] is more recent and relevant because it proposes the anatomic and histologic subdivision of osteomyelitis (medullary, superficial, located, or diffused) and introduces the important concept of host immunocompetence, which is relevant to the onset and diffusion of infections.

Chronic Osteomyelitis After Trauma/Surgery

Chronic osteomyelitis is characterized by a low-grade presentation, with lymphocyte and plasma

Table 1
Mechanisms of radiotracer accumulation in infection and inflammation

Radiotracer	Mechanism
[^{18}F]FDG	Uptake in metabolically active cells including macrophages and leukocytes
^{99m}Tc/^{111}In-labeled autologous WBCs (leukocytes)	Active migration into sites of inflammation
^{99m}Tc-labeled bisphosphonates	Uptake in sites of increased perfusion and extravasation (early phase) and increased bone formation (late phase)
^{67}Ga-citrate	Increased perfusion, extravasation caused by increased vessel permeability, locally binding to lactoferrin
^{99m}Tc-labeled nanocolloids	Uptake in macrophages (inflammation, bone marrow, liver, spleen)
^{99m}Tc/^{111}In-labeled proteins (IgG, albumin)	Extravasation (increased perfusion and vessel permeability)

cell infiltrates and variable degrees of necrosis and osteosclerosis. This definition of chronic osteomyelitis includes patients in whom osteomyelitis is persistent despite adequate therapy or in whom the diagnosis of recurrent bone infection is being considered. The diagnosis is difficult in these patients because chronic bone infection alters the normal anatomy and physiology of bone. These changes and the low-grade presentation make accurate diagnosis difficult. As a result, patients often undergo multiple diagnostic techniques to either confirm or exclude the presence of infection.[22] There is a variety of imaging techniques available for excluding or confirming chronic osteomyelitis, although none seem superior to FDG-PET, because FDG is avidly taken up by activated macrophages, which predominate in the chronic phase of infection.

FDG-PET imaging has been shown to accurately distinguish chronic osteomyelitis from the normal postsurgical or posttraumatic healing process. This finding is in contrast with bone scintigraphy, which may not only be positive in active disease but also in healing bone. Koort and colleagues[25] conducted an experimental animal study to evaluate whether FDG-PET could differentiate between normal bone healing and local osteomyelitis. A localized osteomyelitis model of the rabbit tibia was created, in which 2 groups were formed (an osteomyelitis group [n = 8] and a normal inflammation group [n = 8]). In the normal inflammation group, uncomplicated bone healing was associated with an initial increase in FDG uptake at 3 weeks, which subsequently returned to normal by 6 weeks. Conversely, in the osteomyelitis group, localized infection resulted in continuous intense radiotracer uptake. Therefore, FDG-PET was clearly beneficial in the postsurgical follow-up, because it could identify superimposed infections that arise at some point in the future.[26]

A meta-analysis performed by Termaat and colleagues[22] concluded that FDG-PET has the highest accuracy for confirming or excluding the diagnosis of chronic osteomyelitis. In this meta-analysis, the pooled sensitivity showed that FDG-PET was the most sensitive technique, with a sensitivity of 96% compared with 82% for bone scintigraphy, 61% for radiolabeled WBC scintigraphy, 78% for combined bone and radiolabeled WBC scintigraphy, and 84% for MR imaging. The pooled specificity showed that bone scintigraphy alone has the lowest specificity of 25% compared with 60% for MR imaging, 77% for radiolabeled WBC scintigraphy, 84% for combined bone and radiolabeled WBC scintigraphy, and 91% for FDG-PET (**Fig. 1**).[27] The review also revealed that leukocyte scintigraphy has an appropriate diagnostic accuracy in the peripheral skeleton, but that FDG-PET is superior for detecting chronic osteomyelitis in the axial skeleton.

In the meta-analysis by Termaat and colleagues, MR imaging was sensitive for detecting bone

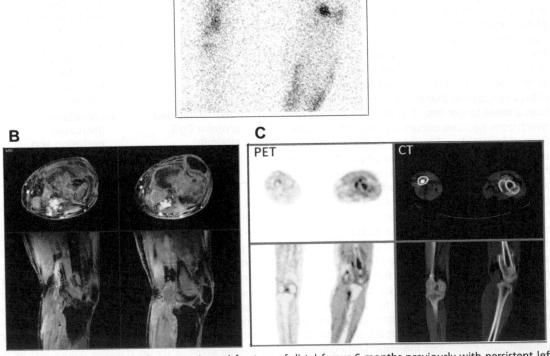

Fig. 1. The patient is status after comminuted fracture of distal femur 6 months previously with persistent left lateral knee pain. (A) Coronal 24-hour ^{111}In-labeled leukocyte image shows focally intense uptake in the left distal femur. (B) Sagittal and axial postcontrast fat-suppressed T1-weighted MR images show an associated rim enhancing fluid collection (*arrows*) and surrounding soft tissue enhancement at the fracture site. (C) Axial and coronal FDG-PET/CT images show increased FDG uptake in the intramedullary distal femur and surrounding soft tissue. Surgical pathology confirmed these findings with bacterial culture showing presence of infection by *Staphylococcus* species (coagulase negative). (*Image courtesy of* Abass Alavi, MD, Hospital of the University of Pennsylvania.)

alterations such as edema (increased signal intensity on T2-weighted images) and increased regional enhancement. However, MR imaging lacks specificity unless clear morphologic signs for osteomyelitis are observed. Another disadvantage of MR imaging is its occasional inability to distinguish infectious from reactive inflammation. MR imaging has a 100% negative predictive value for excluding osteomyelitis. If the marrow is completely normal on all pulse sequences, infection is reliably excluded. The positive predictive value of MR imaging, or its ability to differentiate osteomyelitis from other causes of abnormal marrow signal intensity (such as neuropathic arthropathy and "reactive marrow edema"), is not as high. Reactive marrow edema is noninfectious and can be seen in bone marrow adjacent to a site of soft tissue infection or other focus of osteomyelitis, or can be have other noninfectious causes such as recent contusion. The pathogenesis is unknown but it is thought to represent a type of vasogenic hyperemia. The signal intensity of reactive marrow can mimic that of osteomyelitis and can enhance after contrast administration, producing false-positive results, in which case additional diagnostic procedures are often needed.[18,28]

A retrospective study of patients with a history of fractures or orthopedic interventions compared the results of FDG-PET scans with those of bone scans, radiographs, CT, and MR imaging, as well as surgical pathology. The results of this study revealed that increased FDG uptake did not persist in fractures more than a month after occurrence.[29,30] Thus, on FDG-PET, a history of fracture or surgical trauma is less likely to cause false-positive results in the evaluation for chronic osteomyelitis. Compared with other scintigraphic techniques, FDG-PET is superior for distinguishing soft tissue infection from osteomyelitis.[2,31]

Several studies have shown FDG-PET to be superior to other imaging modalities in the detection of chronic osteomyelitis in the axial skeleton, an area in which leukocyte scintigraphy for imaging chronic osteomyelitis is of limited value. FDG-PET accurately detects spinal osteomyelitis and could potentially replace ^{67}Ga-citrate for this purpose. For example, Guhlmann and colleagues[32] showed that FDG-PET was particularly valuable in detecting osteomyelitis in the axial skeleton in patients with suspected chronic osteomyelitis, in which the labeled WBC method was proved to be ineffective. In addition, a prospective study by Meller and colleagues[5] revealed that, in patients with suspected active chronic osteomyelitis, FDG-PET was superior to ^{111}In-labeled leukocyte imaging in the diagnosis of chronic osteomyelitis

in the central skeleton. Various analyses showed that the sensitivity of leukocyte scintigraphy decreased significantly from 84% for chronic osteomyelitis in the peripheral skeleton to 21% in the axial skeleton.

Most often when leukocyte imaging is considered positive for osteomyelitis, there is an abnormally increased area of radiotracer activity. However, within the axial skeleton (and in particular the spine), osteomyelitis has also been described as appearing as a photopenic or cold lesion. The nonspecific uptake of labeled leukocytes has been suggested to be caused by the presence of hematopoietic bone marrow in the axial skeleton. The appearance of focally decreased uptake of labeled cells in infections of the axial skeleton is poorly understood, but may arise because acute infection is characterized by a neutrophilic response that, over time, is abated and is replaced by a monocyte/macrophage response. Because only 30% to 80% of the reinjected leukocytes are neutrophils and only 2% to 8% are monocytes, there may be too few monocytes present to be successfully imaged. Consequently, increased radiotracer uptake on leukocyte imaging can only be present as long as a sufficient neutrophilic response exists. Because this neutrophilic response (and hence labeled cell activity) subsides, the only evidence that a pathologic process exists is likely to be the photopenic defect. The observed variance in diagnostic accuracy of leukocyte scintigraphy could be explained by the location of chronic osteomyelitis. Leukocyte scintigraphy for chronic osteomyelitis of the axial skeleton was the least sensitive of the imaging techniques. Thus, although leukocyte scintigraphy is an accurate technique for the detection of chronic osteomyelitis in the peripheral skeleton, it is an inappropriate technique for diagnosing chronic osteomyelitis in the axial skeleton.[27]

FDG-PET may have limited value in a diagnosis of uncomplicated cases of acute osteomyelitis compared with the combination of physical examination, evaluation of biochemical marker alteration (WBC count, serum C-reactive protein, and serum erythrocyte sedimentation rate), and 3-phase bone scanning or MR imaging. However, FDG-PET is the most sensitive technique for detecting chronic osteomyelitis and has a greater specificity than leukocyte scintigraphy, ^{67}Ga scintigraphy, bone scintigraphy, or MR imaging.[27]

Even with FDG-PET, there are significant limitations and drawbacks, the major one being its lack of anatomic landmarks, which sometimes makes it difficult to spatially localize sites of radiotracer uptake. However, integrated PET/CT scanners overcome the paucity of anatomic information on

FDG-PET scans. False-positive results in FDG-PET imaging can be caused by postsurgical inflammatory changes for as long as 6 months after the procedure. Thus, it has been proposed that an interval of 3 to 6 months should be allowed before FDG-PET imaging to minimize the risk of false-positive results during stages of postsurgical and traumatic bone healing. However, a negative FDG-PET scan can virtually eliminate the possibility of chronic osteomyelitis.[33]

PROSTHESIS-RELATED OSTEOMYELITIS

Hip replacement is a surgical procedure in which the hip joint is replaced by a prosthetic implant. Hip replacement surgery can be performed as a total replacement or a hemi (half) replacement. Such joint replacement surgery is most often performed to relieve osteoarthritic pain or repair severe physical joint damage as part of hip fracture treatment. Complications after hip arthroplasty are common causes for surgical revision, which can be related to either aseptic loosening of components (loss of fixation) as a result of mechanical failure or, in a smaller percentage of patients, to periprosthetic joint infection. In patients with suspected or confirmed loosening of the prosthesis, the possibility of superimposed infection, which is a serious complication, should be considered in most clinical settings.[2] Pain is common following the implantation of joint prostheses or of metallic devices for fracture, and is a common manifestation of aseptic loosening and infection, such that distinction between these 2 entities is difficult, if not impossible, in most clinical circumstances; however, preoperative differentiation of aseptic loosening from periprosthetic infection is essential for optimal patient care, because these entities are associated with different treatment plans (eg, revision surgery vs long-term intravenous antibiotic therapy followed by surgery).

Radionuclide imaging has been investigated to help differentiate between aseptic loosening and infection in the setting of prostheses. Bone scans were introduced as a potential adjunct in the preoperative work-up for infection, although the specificity was reported as too low for proper confirmation of periprosthetic infection.[34] Conventional ^{99m}Tc sulfur colloid bone marrow scintigraphy is an excellent screening tool to exclude infection.[35] However, the combination of a ^{111}In-labeled leukocyte scan and sulfur colloid bone marrow scintigraphy improves both sensitivity and specificity (Fig. 2A, B).[36] However, these techniques are complex and expensive, require in vitro labeling of the WBC with potential for contamination with pathogens or mixing blood samples among patients, and require at least 24 hours for completion of the procedure. In addition, the low sensitivity and specificity values reported by Scher and colleagues[37] (77% sensitivity, 86% specificity) for assessment of the presence of infection further decreases preference for this approach.

Some investigators have turned to other radiotracers to accurately identify the infected prosthesis without the limitations of leukocyte-sulfur colloid bone marrow scintigraphy. One radiotracer that has aroused considerable interest is FDG.[31] Uptake of this agent depends on glucose metabolism. Activated leukocytes are present in large numbers around both aseptically loosened and infected prostheses, and this circumstance poses a serious obstacle to the success of FDG-PET for evaluation of the painful prosthesis. However, FDG-PET has great potential as a preoperative diagnostic tool that can compensate for some of the pitfalls encountered with routine serology and joint fluid culture during the preoperative work-up. The use of PET is advantageous compared with anatomic imaging modalities because it is not affected by the presence of metal implants used for orthopedic procedures and provides improved

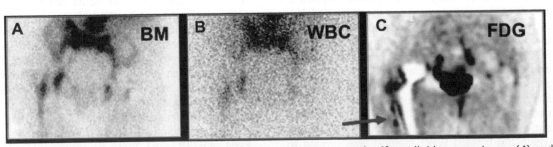

Fig. 2. The patient presented with a painful right hip prosthesis: coronal sulfur colloid marrow image (A) and coronal ^{111}In-labeled leukocyte image (B) show increased radiotracer uptake along the lateral aspect of the right femoral prosthesis with spatial congruence, consistent with absence of infection. (C) Coronal FDG-PET image shows increased FDG uptake at the bone-prosthesis interface along the lateral aspect of the femoral stem, which provides definitive evidence of infection (arrow). Biopsy specimens were positive for osteomyelitis. BM, bone marrow. (Image courtesy of Abass Alavi, MD, Hospital of the University of Pennsylvania.)

spatial resolution relative to conventional nuclear medicine techniques. FDG-PET in patients with the suspicion for total joint replacement infection has shown promising results.[38]

Our group was among the first to use FDG-PET to evaluate arthroplasty-associated infection in a large patient population. In this investigation of 62 patients (36 knee and 38 hip prostheses),[39] the overall sensitivity for the population studied was 90.5% and the specificity was 81.1% in the diagnosis of infected lower limb prostheses.

Reinartz and colleagues[36] studied 92 possibly infected hip prostheses with FDG-PET and reported a sensitivity, specificity, and accuracy of 93.9%, 94.9%, and 94.6%, respectively. Nonspecific FDG uptake after hip arthroplasty can last up to 2 decades in patients without any symptoms.[39] This nonspecific FDG activity is generally located in the regions adjacent to the head and neck of the hip prosthesis and should not be interpreted as a sign of infection. The increased FDG activity caused by periprosthetic infection should be in the periprosthetic soft tissue or arthroplasty interface.[40]

Multiple investigators agree that the establishment of appropriate diagnostic criteria for periprosthetic infection with FDG-PET is critical for optimal use of this technique because interpretation of all sites of increased periprosthetic uptake as positive for infection results in low specificity. In particular, increased FDG activity around the head or neck of the prosthesis is common following arthroplasty and should not be interpreted as suggesting infection.[39] However, increased FDG uptake that is present along the lower portion of the interface between the prosthesis and bone is commonly associated with infection (see **Fig. 2**C). Manthey and colleagues[41] proposed that intense FDG uptake at the bone-prosthesis interface should be reported as positive for infection, whereas an intermediate degree of uptake suggests aseptic loosening, and uptake only in the synovium should be considered as synovitis.

Zhuang and colleagues[38] suggested that the location of increased FDG uptake is the most important factor when this technique is used to diagnose periprosthetic infection in patients who have undergone prior hip arthroplasty. By adopting the standard criterion of presence of FDG between the bone and prosthesis at the level of the midshaft portion of the prosthesis, the accuracy of FDG-PET is substantially increased.[27]

Despite its limitations, combined leukocyte and bone marrow scintigraphy remains the imaging gold standard for the diagnosis of infected joint replacements. Sensitivities and specificities are reported between 86% and 100% and 89% and 94%, respectively.[2] At the present time, there are varying views about the potential of FDG-PET in the evaluation of prostheses. Some investigators think that FDG-PET has excellent sensitivity but poor specificity, whereas other reports indicate that the specificity of FDG-PET is good but the sensitivity is less than optimal. These different conclusions may result from the different interpretation criteria used by these investigators. Thus, it seems that establishment of criteria for diagnosing periprosthetic infections with FDG-PET is critical for optimal use of this method. More studies are needed to define the roles of FDG-PET and to establish criteria for the evaluation of infection prostheses.[2]

VERTEBRAL OSTEOMYELITIS

Spine infections include vertebral osteomyelitis, disc space infections, and epidural abscess. These entities are uncommon, with an incidence of 1 case per 100,000 to 250,000 people per year for vertebral osteomyelitis. Vertebral osteomyelitis represents only 2% to 4% of all cases of osteomyelitis. However, some reviews suggest that the incidence of spinal infection is increasing. This increase may be secondary to increased use of spinal fusion surgery and other forms of instrumentation, as well as to aging of the population. Because of its rarity and vague initial signs and symptoms, diagnosis is often delayed.

Vertebral osteomyelitis can result from hematogenous seeding, direct inoculation at the time of spinal surgery or penetrating trauma, or from contiguous spread from an infection in the adjacent soft tissue. In the postoperative spine, direct inoculation of pathogens into the traumatized subcutaneous tissues and intervertebral disc space, through the posterior route, is thought to be the major route of infection.[42,43] Postoperative spinal infection is typically the result of bacterial seeding in the surgical field, followed by a latent period with activation at a later time. Direct extension of contiguous infection into the vertebrae and discs can be caused by many sources of infection; for instance, extension from a retropharyngeal abscess or a retroperitoneal abscess may result in osteomyelitis and discitis. In addition, direct extension from compartments surrounding the spine may result in additional infections, such as paravertebral, epidural, or psoas abscesses.

Staphylococcus aureus is the most common microorganism implicated in pyogenic vertebral osteomyelitis, followed by *Escherichia coli*.[44] Coagulase-negative staphylococci and *Propionibacterium acnes* are the organisms that are most often the cause of exogenous osteomyelitis after spinal surgery, particularly if fixation devices are used.[44–46] However, in the case of prolonged bacteremia (eg, infection associated with pacemaker electrodes), hematogenous vertebral osteomyelitis caused by low-virulence microorganisms (eg, coagulase-negative staphylococci) has been described.[44,47] Most patients with hematogenous pyogenic vertebral osteomyelitis have underlying medical issues, including diabetes mellitus, coronary artery disease, immunosuppressive disorders, cancer, or chronic renal failure requiring hemodialysis.[48]

Approximately 90% to 95% of pyogenic spinal infections are confined to the vertebral body and intervertebral disc, whereas only 5% to 10% of cases involve the posterior elements of the spine. This disparity has been attributed in part to the voluminous blood supply to the vertebral body and its rich, cellular marrow. Bacteria circulating through the blood may enter a vertebra or a disc space via its arterial blood supply or via the venous system. In the typical case, bacteria enter the vertebral body through small arteries arising from larger periosteal arteries that, in turn, branch from the spinal arteries. In adults, blockage of these small arteries by septic emboli may lead to infarction of large amounts of bone. Subsequently, bacteria can readily colonize a large bony sequestrum adjacent to the disc. After bacterial colonization, bacteria originating from the endplate region may secondarily invade the avascular disc.

Back pain is the most common presenting symptom of vertebral osteomyelitis, and fever is not always present. The location of the pain depends on the site of infection, although the differential diagnosis of back pain is broad. As a result of the nonspecific nature of many signs and symptoms of vertebral osteomyelitis and the frequent absence of fever, there is often a delay between the onset of symptoms and diagnosis (range of 42–59 days in 5 studies).[44] Thus, most patients have prolonged symptoms before diagnosis.

Prompt diagnosis can be facilitated by early appropriate imaging techniques together with bacteriologic culture and histopathology, which are crucial for determining treatment. Adequate treatment shortens the duration of the infection and reduces the likelihood of severe complications, such as neurologic compromise.[19] Blood cultures are of particular importance in the evaluation of vertebral osteomyelitis. A positive culture precludes the need for more invasive procedures, although in vertebral osteomyelitis it is common for blood cultures and biopsy specimens to remain negative, in which case the clinical and noninvasive imaging findings become paramount in diagnosing spinal infections and assessing response to treatment.

If left untreated, vertebral osteomyelitis (and other spinal infections) can lead to permanent paralysis, significant spinal deformity, or death. It can result in severe compression of the neural structures because of the formation of an epidural abscess or because of a pathologic fracture resulting from bone softening. Thus imaging is critical to localizing infection and identifying pyogenic complications, such as an epidural, paravertebral, or disc space abscess.

Plain film radiographs are often obtained as an initial diagnostic test, because they are widely available and may reveal an alternative diagnosis (eg, bone metastasis or osteoporotic compression fracture); however, radiography is not a sensitive test for osteomyelitis. In patients with neurologic impairment, MR imaging should be the first diagnostic step in assessing for potential spinal epidural abscess and excluding a herniated disc.

MR imaging, with an accuracy of 90%, is the diagnostic imaging procedure of choice for vertebral osteomyelitis, because it permits early diagnosis of infection and provides direct visualization of the spinal cord, subarachnoid space, extradural soft tissues, and spinal column without the use of intrathecal contrast material. Modic and colleagues[49] reported MR imaging to be 96% sensitive and 92% specific for the diagnosis of vertebral osteomyelitis, with a 100% negative predictive value, although the positive predictive value to differentiate osteomyelitis from other causes of abnormal marrow signal is not as high. Acute vertebral osteomyelitis on MR imaging can be identified as early as 1 to 2 days after infection, which is reflected by bone marrow edema with decreased signal intensity on T1-weighted images and increased signal intensity on fat-suppressed T2-weighted images. Gadolinium enhanced T1-weighted images also provide clear delineation of the spinal cord, epidural space, subarachnoid space, extradural soft tissues, and paraspinal soft tissues to assess associated complications. Even with the aforementioned advantages of MR imaging, limitations still exist. MR imaging relies on structural changes for diagnosis, although, in postsurgical situations in which the normal anatomy is altered or susceptibility artifacts are present, this technique becomes less reliable.[50] Furthermore, MR imaging is sensitive to motion artifacts, so that patients with movement disorders may not be suitable candidates for this study. In addition, patients with pacemakers and cardiac valves may not be eligible for MR imaging. FDG-PET or bone ^{67}Ga scintigraphy imaging can be a useful alternative if MR imaging cannot be performed or is not diagnostic based on the limitations described earlier.[19]

MR imaging is more sensitive than CT for the early detection of osteomyelitis, and therefore CT is generally indicated only if the patient has a contraindication to MR imaging or if CT is needed to guide a percutaneous biopsy. Neither CT nor MR imaging has 100% specificity; the diagnosis that is most difficult to differentiate from vertebral osteomyelitis on imaging studies is erosive osteochondrosis, because its features may mimic those of vertebral osteomyelitis.

The structural imaging techniques described earlier are frequently used in patients with suspected spinal infection. However, these approaches are sometimes nonspecific, and difficulties in differentiating infectious from degenerative or postoperative changes can arise. Although MR imaging cannot always distinguish osteomyelitis from severe degenerative arthritis, with the edemalike granulation changes within the vertebral endplates, molecular imaging studies such as FDG-PET and ^{67}Ga scintigraphy may be useful, thus improving diagnostic accuracy.

Bone scintigraphy is widely available, easily performed, and rapidly completed. The results can be positive as early as 2 days after the onset of symptoms. Gratz and colleagues[19] prospectively studied 30 patients with vertebral osteomyelitis and reported that bone scintigraphy was 86% sensitive for diagnosing spinal osteomyelitis, and that could be increased to 92% by performing SPECT. Although sensitive, bone scintigraphy is not specific. In addition, 3-phase bone scintigraphy and analysis of uptake patterns have been used to enhance the accuracy of bone scintigraphy for diagnosing spinal osteomyelitis. Love and colleagues[51] found that the specificity was improved with the 3-phase technique, at the expense of sensitivity, which in their series decreased from 92% to 36%. With respect to uptake patterns, investigators found that abnormal uptake in 2 contiguous vertebrae on SPECT was the single most accurate criterion (71%) for detecting spinal osteomyelitis, although it was still suboptimal in diagnostic performance.[52]

Other limitations to bone scintigraphy include false-negative results, which have been reported in elderly patients with spinal osteomyelitis, likely caused by regional ischemia secondary to atherosclerotic disease. Radiotracer uptake may also persist after infection has resolved, because of bone remodeling and repair. Vertebral osteomyelitis is often accompanied, and at times may be mimicked, by soft tissue infection. Bone scintigraphy is not sensitive for detecting soft tissue infections and consequently cannot be the sole radionuclide test performed in patients with suspected spinal osteomyelitis.[19]

For osteomyelitis, ^{67}Ga scintigraphy is usually performed with bone scintigraphy. [67]Ga scintigraphy improves the specificity of bone scintigraphy,

detects infection earlier than bone scintigraphy alone, and identifies the presence of accompanying soft tissue infection. The current radionuclide imaging method of choice for diagnosing spinal osteomyelitis is combined bone gallium scintigraphy, with reported results that are comparable to those of MR imaging.[53] In addition to enhancing the specificity of the bone scintigraphy, ^{67}Ga scintigraphy is useful for detecting abscesses that may accompany vertebral osteomyelitis. There are data that indicate that ^{67}Ga SPECT is comparable with combined bone gallium imaging for diagnosis of this entity.[54] Regardless of whether ^{67}Ga imaging is performed alone or in combination with bone scintigraphy, the suboptimal imaging characteristics of ^{67}Ga and the need for 2 isotopes with multiple imaging sessions over several days are disadvantages to this approach. Moreover, there is nothing specific about ^{67}Ga uptake in infection because it also accumulates in other conditions, including primary and metastatic neoplasms, and in aseptic inflammation and traumatic foci. There are few data available on its use in postoperative vertebral osteomyelitis, although several investigators have reported increased radiotracer accumulation in normally healing surgical sites for up to several months after surgery. Uptake in postoperative inflammation without superimposed osteomyelitis has also been described. Despite these limitations, ^{67}Ga scintigraphy is probably superior to bone scintigraphy in the follow-up of infection, as well as for monitoring of therapeutic response because it is less sensitive to bone remodeling and more accurately reflects the degree of activity in the infectious process.[19]

As previously mentioned, in vertebral (axial skeleton) osteomyelitis, WBC imaging has low sensitivity, approximately 50%, which has been hypothesized to reflect the inability of leukocytes to migrate into the encapsulated infection.[55] This inability may cause photopenic lesions, which are not specific for infection and, together with the physiologic uptake of WBCs into the bone marrow, hinders accurate detection of vertebral infection. However, leukocyte images are typically interpreted as positive for infection when the area of interest shows increased activity relative to some reference point. In the absence of infection, leukocytes are generally not incorporated into areas of increased bone mineral turnover, thus making leukocyte imaging highly specific for the diagnosis of osteomyelitis. This test is especially valuable in the setting of underlying osseous disorders such as trauma, tumor, and other conditions that limit the usefulness of routine bone scintigraphy.

The conventional radionuclide tests discussed earlier have mostly been replaced by MR imaging. FDG-PET has a diagnostic accuracy similar to that of MR imaging in patients with osteomyelitis and is preferable when a patient has metallic implants. FDG-PET has been shown to have a high sensitivity of at least 95%, with high specificities of more than 87%. Gratz and colleagues[56] showed that FDG-PET was superior to MR imaging in patients who had a history of prior surgery, in those who had high-grade infection with paravertebral abscess, and in low-grade spondylitis and discitis. De Winter and colleagues[57] investigated FDG-PET in 57 patients, including 27 with metallic hardware, suspected of having spinal infection after previous spinal surgery. Twenty-six percent of patients had vertebral osteomyelitis, and infection was present in 37% of patients with hardware and in 17% of patients without hardware. Using the optimal maximum threshold standardized uptake values (SUVs), the sensitivity, specificity, and accuracy of FDG-PET were 100%, 81%, and 86%, respectively. The positive predictive value was 65%, and the negative predictive value was 100%. Among those without metallic hardware, there were 2 false-positive scans, both in patients who had undergone surgery within 6 months before imaging. Among patients with metallic hardware, there were 6 false-positive results, which were not related to recent surgery. The cause of false-positive results could be established in only 1 case: instability of the hardware. The sensitivity, specificity, and accuracy were not significantly different between subgroups of patients who had surgery less than, versus more than, 6 months before FDG-PET. The specificity was 65% in the group with metallic hardware and 92% in the group without metallic hardware. In 60% of patients, infection was excluded with FDG-PET. The investigators concluded that

chronic postoperative spinal infection can be excluded when FDG-PET is negative. The overall accuracy of FDG-PET in this prospective study was good (86%), with a negative predictive value of 100%. Although specificity is suboptimal, comparable diagnostic performance is not achievable with bone scintigraphy, leukocyte scintigraphy, or MR imaging.[19,58]

As described in the published results, a negative FDG-PET scan excludes vertebral osteomyelitis with a high degree of certainty. The specificity of the test is acceptable, although caution should be used in interpreting a positive PET study, particularly in the presence of metallic hardware.[19] A general limitation of FDG-PET is that, despite high contrast resolution, the anatomic information available remains limited. To improve this, integrated PET/CT in-line systems have recently been introduced that provide coregistered PET and CT images. The more precise localization of FDG activity obtained with such combined systems further enhances the use of PET in those indications (**Fig. 3**).[19]

De Winter and colleagues[57] were able to show that the specificity for spinal infection decreased to 75% only if patients had undergone surgery less than 6 months before PET and to 65% if osteosynthetic material was present. However, because MR imaging is prone to susceptibility artifacts when metallic hardware is present, FDG-PET is currently the most sensitive imaging modality in the evaluation of such patients.[59] Furthermore, in cases of severe degenerative disease with edema-like changes in the endplates and adjacent discs, MR imaging can give false-positive results.[60]

Although most of the published series are small, FDG-PET seems to be superior for the detection of vertebral osteomyelitis and in the differentiation of degenerative from infectious discitis, compared with ^{67}Ga imaging or MR imaging.[61] PET is highly

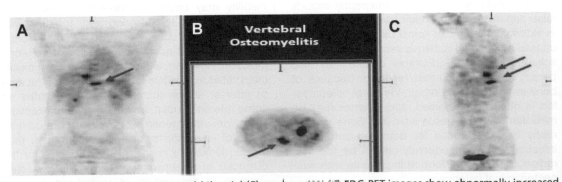

Fig. 3. Patient with back pain. Coronal (A), axial (B), and sagittal (C) FDG-PET images show abnormally increased FDG uptake (arrows) in 2 adjacent vertebrae within the thoracic spine, in keeping with vertebral osteomyelitis. (*From* Zhuang H, Alavi A. 18-fluorodeoxyglucose positron emission tomographic imaging in the detection and monitoring of infection and inflammation. Semin Nucl Med 2002;32(1):47–59; with permission, **Fig. 1.**)

sensitive, is completed in a single session, and has image resolution superior to that obtained with SPECT. Although FDG uptake in noninfected fractures may normalize more rapidly than gallium or diphosphonate uptake, differentiation of infection from tumor may still be problematic. Furthermore, inflammatory reactions incited by metallic hardware may also adversely affect specificity.[62] Nevertheless, there is an increasing body of evidence that supports the use of FDG-PET/CT for diagnosis of spinal infection, especially in patients with contraindications to MR imaging, as well as in the postoperative spine. With the rapid evolution and proliferation of in-line PET/CT and SPECT/CT systems, well-designed prospective comparisons of FDG-PET/CT and ^{67}Ga SPECT/CT should be undertaken to validate these initial observations and to determine the potential of each of these radiotracers and associated imaging techniques for monitoring response to treatment.[19]

DIABETIC FOOT INFECTION AND CHARCOT OSTEOARTHROPATHY

Diabetes mellitus affects about 5% of the US population, and each year more than 10% of diabetic patients are hospitalized for foot complications from the disease, which are the principal cause of morbidity and mortality in this population.[51] Foot infections and their sequelae are among the most common and severe complications of diabetes mellitus. Foot infections are a major contributing factor to diabetes being the leading cause of nontraumatic lower extremity amputations in the United States. The major predisposing factor to infection in the diabetic foot is the neuropathic ulcer, which results from trauma or excessive pressure on a foot that lacks protective sensation. Once the cutaneous integument is breached, the ulcer may serve as a portal of entry for microorganisms, becoming actively infected and, by contiguous extension, involving deeper tissues, including bone, which may lead to frank osteomyelitis. These ulcers are associated with more than 90% of diabetic pedal osteomyelitis cases.[9]

Early diagnosis of osteomyelitis in the diabetic foot is crucial because antibiotic therapy can be curative and may prevent amputation. However, the clinical presentation of osteomyelitis is frequently insidious, because roughly two-thirds of diabetic patients with complicated pedal ulcers present without systemic illness, further complicating and obscuring the clinical picture of deep-seated infection. Although the isolation of bacteria from a bone biopsy together with histologic findings of inflammatory cells and osteonecrosis is considered the reference standard for detecting

osteomyelitis, this option has risks in diabetic patients, because the procedure may inadvertently induce osteomyelitis or necrosis of the bone. Furthermore, an underlying neurodegenerative osteoarthropathy can mislead clinicians and lead to a delay in diagnosis. As a result of these complications, as well as the difficulty in detecting deep-seated infections, imaging studies are often needed to confirm the biopsy diagnosis.[27]

Neuropathic (Charcot) osteoarthropathy is a rare phenomenon, making it difficult for clinicians to recognize, although it is the main disease entity that leads to a delay in diagnosis. It is estimated that the overall prevalence of the Charcot foot in the general diabetic population varies between 0.1% and 7.5%. However, diabetic patients with peripheral neuropathy develop Charcot foot at a rate of 29% to 35%. However, if not recognized, Charcot foot may lead to progressive foot deformity, ulceration, or osteomyelitis, and eventually amputation.

Location is a guiding feature for diagnosis: osteomyelitis is predisposed to occur at pressure points and areas of ulceration along bony protuberances. Consequently, the most common locations for osteomyelitis are at the metatarsal heads and interphalangeal joints in the forefoot, at the distal fibula, and at the plantar aspect of the posterior calcaneus of the hindfoot. In Charcot arthropathy, the tarsal and tarsometatarsal joints are affected in 60% (**Fig. 4**A–C), the metatarsophalangeal joints in 30%, and the tibiotalar joint in about 10% of cases. Repetitive stress on an insensitive foot leads to bone and joint disruption, deformity, and instability, which in turn leads to degeneration, subluxation, and eventually destruction of the joint. The repetitive cycle of injury, destruction, incomplete healing, and partial repair results in a grossly deformed foot. The longitudinal arch of the foot collapses, producing the so-called rocker bottom appearance. Clinically, the neuropathic joint usually presents like osteomyelitis, with swelling that can be massive, crepitus (caused by destruction of bone and cartilage), instability (caused by loss of the longitudinal arch), palpable loose bodies, and large osteophytes. Pain is often absent but, when present, is typically not proportional to the gross appearance of the foot. Synovial effusions are usually noninflammatory or hemorrhagic and are composed predominantly of mononuclear cells.[63] Although infection is not a common complication of the neuropathic joint, differentiation between the 2 entities or diagnosing infection superimposed on the neuropathic joint is challenging, especially because osteomyelitis of the foot is a condition that necessitates early identification and intervention to prevent amputation of the lower extremity.

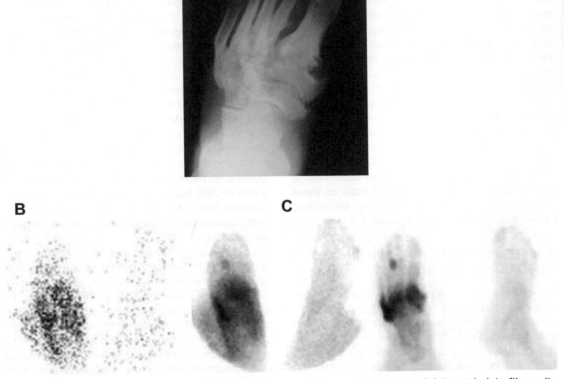

Fig. 4. Diabetic patient with prior partial foot amputation presents with foot pain. (*A*) Frontal plain film radiograph of the foot shows extensive tarsal and metatarsal joint destruction with marked soft tissue swelling, in keeping with a neuropathic (Charcot) osteoarthropathy. The fifth digit phalanges and distal metatarsal were previously amputated. (*B, C*) Coronal 3-phase bone scintigraphic images are positive. (*From* Palestro CJ, Love C. Nuclear medicine and diabetic foot infections. Semin Nucl Med 2009;391:52–65; with permission, **Fig. 6.**)

Because it is inexpensive and available widely, plain film radiography is usually the initial imaging study used to evaluate patients suspected of having a complicated diabetic foot ulcer. Positive study is used to evaluate patients suspected of having a complicated diabetic foot ulcer. Positive findings for infection on plain film radiography may include the presence of soft tissue gas, cortical destruction (**Fig. 5**), periosteal reaction, and osteopenia, although these changes may not be visible until 2 to 4 weeks after the onset of infection, which accounts for its poor sensitivity.

In addition, the diagnosis of osteomyelitis is complicated by the observation that acute neurodegenerative osteoarthropathy can present with symptoms, signs, and imaging findings similar to those of infection, thus compromising the specificity of plain film radiography. Thus, although plain film radiography is a simple and inexpensive

screening modality, its overall low sensitivity often results in a delay in diagnosis, adversely affecting the management of patients if used as the sole diagnostic test (see **Fig. 5**).[64]

With such extensive bony changes, 3-phase bone scintigraphy is usually positive (see **Fig. 4**B), regardless of the presence of infection.[65] The specificity of the 3-phase bone scintigraphy is poor in the setting of any preexisting osseous conditions that cause bone turnover, including neuropathic osteoarthropathy and healing infections. Thus, bone scintigraphy is likely to be helpful only when suspected osteomyelitis is not superimposed on another process that may cause bone remodeling.

Unlike bone scintigraphy, ^{111}In-labeled leukocytes are not incorporated into areas of active bone turnover. However, they do accumulate in both infected and noninfected neuropathic joints. In the past, such uptake was attributed to the

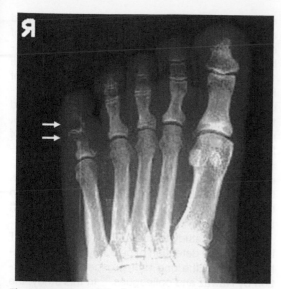

Fig. 5. Patient with foot pain with osteomyelitis. Frontal plain film radiograph shows cortical destruction of phalanges of fifth digit along with soft tissue swelling (*arrows*), characteristic of acute osteomyelitis. (*From* Palestro CJ, Love C. Nuclear medicine and diabetic foot infections. Semin Nucl Med 2009;39: 52–65; with permission, **Fig. 1**.)

inflammation, fractures, and reparative processes that are all parts of the disease. It is now known that labeled leukocyte accumulation in the noninfected neuropathic joint is caused, at least in part, by hematopoietically active bone marrow within the feet.[63] The conversion of fatty marrow into hematopoietically active marrow in induced arthritis of the lower extremities is well documented in animal models, and a similar process may take place in the neuropathic joint. Fractures are an integral part of the neuropathic joint, and

bone marrow is intimately involved in fracture repair, which also may account for the presence of bone marrow in the neuropathic joint. Regardless of the underlying mechanisms, labeled leukocyte accumulation in the noninfected neuropathic joint does occur. As with other sites in the skeleton, performing complementary bone marrow imaging facilitates the differentiation of labeled leukocyte uptake caused by bone marrow from that caused by infection. The sensitivity of the test, when ^{111}In-labeled leukocytes are used, ranges from 72% to 100% and the specificity ranges from 67% to 100%.[63] Thus, combined bone ^{99m}Tc sulfur colloid bone marrow imaging and ^{111}In leukocyte scintigraphy can more accurately differentiate the neuropathic joint from infection (**Fig. 6**).

MR imaging is an effective modality for the evaluation of osteomyelitis involving the feet of diabetic patients, with sensitivity values ranging from 77% to 100%, in the absence of other potential complications, as described later. MR imaging has a significant advantage compared with other techniques for providing excellent spatial resolution and precise anatomic localization of abnormal sites. However, diagnosis of osteomyelitis with MR imaging is often complicated because other processes in the diabetic foot, including neuropathic osteoarthropathy, postsurgical change, and posttraumatic effects, as well as biomechanical stress, can cause changes in the bone marrow or soft tissue similar to those that occur with osteomyelitis. Thus, differentiation between osteomyelitis and neuropathic osteoarthropathy on MR imaging is sometimes difficult because signal alterations caused by edema often have nonspecific causes. As a result, in such settings, the suboptimal specificity of MR imaging for osteomyelitis poses a major challenge for optimal management of these

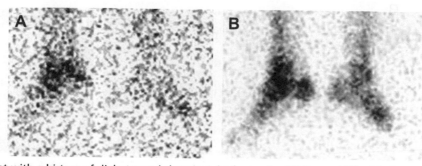

Fig. 6. Patient with a history of diabetes and chronic right foot pain. (*A*) Coronal ^{111}In-labeled WBC image with increased radiotracer activity in the neuropathic joint on the right. (*B*) Coronal ^{99m}Tc sulfur colloid bone marrow image also shows increased radiotracer activity in a distribution similar to that of the labeled WBC study, confirming that the labeled WBC activity is caused by the presence of bone marrow and not infection. Combined leukocyte-marrow scintigraphy was able to accurately differentiate this patient's neuropathic joint from infection. (*From* Palestro CJ, Love C. Nuclear medicine and diabetic foot infections. Semin Nucl Med 2009;39:52–65; with permission, **Fig. 7**.)

patients.[66] However, preliminary data provide evidence of an important role for FDG-PET imaging in assessment of complicated and uncomplicated cases.

In a prospective study that included 39 patients with Charcot osteoarthropathy confirmed at surgery, Höpfner and colleagues[67] noted that FDG-PET with a dedicated full ring PET scanner had a sensitivity of 95%, compared with a coincidence PET camera with a sensitivity of 77%, and MR imaging with a sensitivity of 79%.[68] The investigators noted that FDG-PET can provide an accurate assessment of patients with metal implants, which may otherwise limit evaluation by MR imaging, and that FDG-PET can correctly distinguish osteomyelitis from Charcot foot, soft tissue infection, or septic arthritis.[40,68] FDG-PET provides the surgeon with important additional information for patient management that often is unavailable from MR imaging. As such, FDG-PET may be a useful adjunct in the preoperative evaluation of patients.[67]

Results from our own institution, reported by Basu and colleagues,[69] have been encouraging in the use of FDG-PET for the diagnosis of osteomyelitis in the diabetic foot. In this study, a total of 63 patients, in 4 groups, were evaluated. A low degree of diffuse FDG uptake that was clearly distinguishable from normal joints was observed in the joints of patients with Charcot osteoarthropathy. The maximum SUV in patients with Charcot osteoarthropathy ranged from 0.7 to 2.4 (mean 1.3 ± 0.4), whereas those of midfoot of the healthy control subjects and in the uncomplicated diabetic foot ranged from 0.2 to 0.7 (mean 0.42 ± 0.12) and 0.2 to 0.8 (mean 0.5 ± 0.16), respectively. The only patient with Charcot osteoarthropathy with

superimposed osteomyelitis in this series had a maximum SUV of 6.5, and maximum SUV of sites of osteomyelitis as a complication of the diabetic foot ranged from 2.9 to 6.2 (mean 4.38 ± 1.39). The overall sensitivity and accuracy of FDG-PET in the diagnosis of Charcot osteoarthropathy were 100% and 93.8%, respectively, and those for MR imaging were 76.9% and 75%, respectively. These results indicate the value of FDG-PET in the setting of Charcot osteoarthropathy to allow for reliable differentiation from osteomyelitis whether or not foot ulceration is present. Overall, FDG-PET can differentiate between Charcot neuroarthropathy, osteomyelitis, and soft tissue infection.[68]

The largest study to date of the role of FDG-PET imaging in the detection of osteomyelitis in the diabetic foot was the long-term prospective investigation by Nawaz and colleagues.[66] In this study, the investigators compared the usefulness of FDG-PET with MR imaging as well as with plain film radiographs. Unlike MR imaging, FDG-PET retains a high specificity even in the presence of other coexistent disease in the foot. In addition, initial analysis suggests that, on average, SUVs in regions of sterile inflammation of the Charcot foot tend to occur in the midfoot and are lower than those in the infected sites classically located in the toes or calcaneus subjacent to an ulcer. Quantification of radiotracer activity using maximum SUVs may potentially help to differentiate areas of infection from those of inflammation. The maximum SUV in Charcot foot varied from 0.7 to 2.4 (mean 1.3 ± 0.4), whereas those of osteomyelitis as a complication of the diabetic foot were 2.9 to 6.2 (mean 4.38 ± 1.39) (**Fig. 7**), which supports the usefulness of FDG-PET in the setting of

A   **B**

Coronal Transaxial

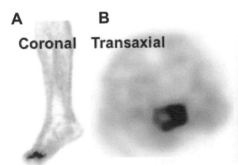
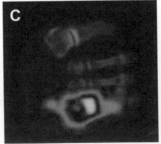
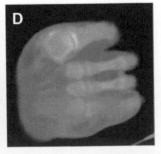

Fig. 7. Diabetic patient with nonhealing wound in the right forefoot, undergoing imaging evaluation for osteomyelitis. Coronal (A) and axial (B) FDG-PET images through the foot show increased FDG uptake in lateral forefoot. (C) Coronal PET/CT fused image localizes abnormal FDG uptake to the base of the fourth metatarsal. (D) Coronal CT image shows mild osteopenia but no gross lytic destruction in the corresponding area. Osteomyelitis was subsequently confirmed by biopsy and microbiological evaluation. (*Reprinted with permission the Society of Nuclear Medicine from:* Keidar Z, Militianu D, Melamed E, et al. The diabetic foot: initial experience with 18F-FDG PET/CT. J Nucl Med 2005;46(3):444–9.)

Charcot neuroarthropathy.[27] Overall, FDG-PET is a highly specific imaging modality for excluding osteomyelitis in the diabetic foot, and is a useful complementary imaging modality, particularly in cases with equivocal MR imaging findings. In addition, in clinical scenarios in which MR imaging is not recommended or possible, the sensitivity and specificity of FDG-PET allow it to be used as the major imaging alternative.[27]

These reports confirm that FDG-PET is useful in the diagnosis of acute infections and is an accurate imaging modality to exclude the diagnosis of osteomyelitis. MR imaging provides precise anatomic detail, but its low specificity to diagnose osteomyelitis in the diabetic foot is predominantly attributed to its inability to distinguish between noninfected bone marrow edema and infection. Hence, the use of MR imaging for evaluation of the diabetic foot, both because of the high sensitivity and its ability to accurately show lesion location and relationships to adjacent structures, is still warranted after plain film radiography with suspicious findings. A positive result on MR imaging may warrant follow-up with FDG-PET imaging because of the improved specificity of the latter imaging technique. With a combined MR imaging and PET imaging protocol, particularly when hybrid PET/MR imaging scanners become clinically available, the management of patients with a complicated diabetic foot may be one of the few clinical scenarios in which there is a significant improvement when using combined dual imaging modalities compared with individual imaging techniques alone.[70]

SUMMARY

Molecular imaging techniques, including FDG-PET, provide improvements in sensitivity and specificity relative to conventional diagnostic techniques alone for the diagnosis of osteomyelitis. The desire to characterize infectious disorders to the fullest extent is expected to result in even greater importance for hybrid multimodality imaging approaches that take advantage of the strengths of existing structural and molecular imaging technologies. To understand how molecular imaging may play a role in the care and treatment of osteomyelitis, it is important to identify unmet diagnostic needs. These needs include the need for (1) more accurate infection detection, (2) earlier and more predictive assessment of therapeutic response, and (3) better characterization of infection/inflammation biology for directing the choice and aggressiveness of therapy for individual patients.

REFERENCES

1. Kaim AH, Gross T, von Schulthess GK. Imaging of chronic posttraumatic osteomyelitis. Eur Radiol 2002;12:1193–202.
2. El-Haddad G, Zhuang H, Gupta N, et al. Evolving role of positron emission tomography in the management of patients with inflammatory and other benign disorders. Semin Nucl Med 2004;34:313–29.
3. Becker W. [The diagnostic potentials of nuclear medicine in chronic infections]. Radiologe 2000;40: 561–7 [in German].
4. Gotthardt M, Bleeker-Rovers CP, Boerman OC, et al. Imaging of inflammation by PET, conventional scintigraphy, and other imaging techniques. J Nucl Med 2010;51:1937–49.
5. Meller J, Koster G, Liersch T, et al. Chronic bacterial osteomyelitis: prospective comparison of (18)F-FDG imaging with a dual-head coincidence camera and (111)In-labelled autologous leucocyte scintigraphy. Eur J Nucl Med Mol Imaging 2002;29:53–60.
6. Hartshorne MF, Graham G, Lancaster J, et al. Gallium-67/technetium-99m methylene diphosphonate ratio imaging: early rabbit osteomyelitis and fracture. J Nucl Med 1985;26:272–7.
7. Hakim SG, Bruecker CW, Jacobsen H, et al. The value of FDG-PET and bone scintigraphy with SPECT in the primary diagnosis and follow-up of patients with chronic osteomyelitis of the mandible. Int J Oral Maxillofac Surg 2006;35:809–16.
8. Horger M, Eschmann SM, Pfannenberg C, et al. Added value of SPECT/CT in patients suspected of having bone infection: preliminary results. Arch Orthop Trauma Surg 2007;127:211–21.
9. Palestro CJ, Love C. Radionuclide imaging of musculoskeletal infection: conventional agents. Semin Musculoskelet Radiol 2007;11:335–52.
10. Strobel K, Stumpe KD. PET/CT in musculoskeletal infection. Semin Musculoskelet Radiol 2007;11:353–64.
11. Kolindou A, Liu Y, Ozker K, et al. In-111 WBC imaging of osteomyelitis in patients with underlying bone scan abnormalities. Clin Nucl Med 1996;21:183–91.
12. Filippi L, Schillaci O. Usefulness of hybrid SPECT/CT in 99mTc-HMPAO-labeled leukocyte scintigraphy for bone and joint infections. J Nucl Med 2006;47: 1908–13.
13. Seabold JE, Nepola JV. Imaging techniques for evaluation of postoperative orthopedic infections. Q J Nucl Med 1999;43:21–8.
14. Datz FL. Indium-111-labeled leukocytes for the detection of infection: current status. Semin Nucl Med 1994;24:92–109.
15. Peterson TE, Manning HC. Molecular imaging: 18F-FDG PET and a whole lot more. J Nucl Med Technol 2009;37:151–61.
16. Kubota R, Yamada S, Kubota K, et al. Intratumoral distribution of luorine-18-fluorodeoxyglucose

in vivo: high accumulation in macrophages and granulation tissues studied by microautoradiography. J Nucl Med 1992;33:1972–80.

17. Pauwels EK, Ribeiro MJ, Stoot JH, et al. FDG accumulation and tumor biology. Nucl Med Biol 1998;25: 317–22.

18. Palestro CJ, Love C, Miller TT. Infection and musculoskeletal conditions: imaging of musculoskeletal infections. Best Pract Res Clin Rheumatol 2006;20: 1197–218.

19. Gemmel F, Dumarey N, Palestro CJ. Radionuclide imaging of spinal infections. Eur J Nucl Med Mol Imaging 2006;33:1226–37.

20. Weiland AJ, Moore JR, Daniel RK. The efficacy of free tissue transfer in the treatment of osteomyelitis. J Bone Joint Surg Am 1984;66:181–93.

21. Schauwecker DS. Osteomyelitis: diagnosis with In-111-labeled leukocytes. Radiology 1989;171:141–6.

22. Termaat MF, Raijmakers PG, Scholten HJ, et al. The accuracy of diagnostic imaging for the assessment of chronic osteomyelitis: a systematic review and meta-analysis. J Bone Joint Surg Am 2005;87:2464–71.

23. Waldvogel FA, Medoff G, Swartz MN. Osteomyelitis: a review of clinical features, therapeutic considerations and unusual aspects. N Engl J Med 1970;282:198–206.

24. Cierny G 3rd, Mader JT, Penninck JJ. A clinical staging system for adult osteomyelitis. Clin Orthop Relat Res 2003;(414):7–24.

25. Koort JK, Makinen TJ, Knuuti J, et al. Comparative 18F-FDG PET of experimental *Staphylococcus aureus* osteomyelitis and normal bone healing. J Nucl Med 2004;45:1406–11.

26. Kumar R. Assessment of therapy response in malignant tumours with 18F-fluorothymidine. Eur J Nucl Med Mol Imaging 2007;34:1334–8.

27. Basu S, Chryssikos T, Moghadam-Kia S, et al. Positron emission tomography as a diagnostic tool in infection: present role and future possibilities. Semin Nucl Med 2009;39:36–51.

28. Craig JG, Amin MB, Wu K, et al. Osteomyelitis of the diabetic foot: MR imaging-pathologic correlation. Radiology 1997;203:849–55.

29. Schmitz A, Risse JH, Textor J, et al. FDG-PET findings of vertebral compression fractures in osteoporosis: preliminary results. Osteoporos Int 2002;13:755–61.

30. Zhuang H, Sam JW, Chacko TK, et al. Rapid normalization of osseous FDG uptake following traumatic or surgical fractures. Eur J Nucl Med Mol Imaging 2003;30:1096–103.

31. Chacko TK, Zhuang H, Stevenson K, et al. The importance of the location of fluorodeoxyglucose uptake in periprosthetic infection in painful hip prostheses. Nucl Med Commun 2002;23:851–5.

32. Guhlmann A, Brecht-Krauss D, Suger G, et al. Chronic osteomyelitis: detection with FDG PET and correlation with histopathologic findings. Radiology 1998;206:749–54.

33. Zhuang H, Duarte PS, Pourdehand M, et al. Exclusion of chronic osteomyelitis with F-18 fluorodeoxyglucose positron emission tomographic imaging. Clin Nucl Med 2000;25:281–4.

34. Levitsky KA, Hozack WJ, Balderston RA, et al. Evaluation of the painful prosthetic joint. Relative value of bone scan, sedimentation rate, and joint aspiration. J Arthroplasty 1991;6:237–44.

35. Chryssikos T, Parvizi J, Ghanem E, et al. FDG-PET imaging can diagnose periprosthetic infection of the hip. Clin Orthop Relat Res 2008;466:1338–42.

36. Reinartz P, Mumme T, Hermanns B, et al. Radionuclide imaging of the painful hip arthroplasty: positron-emission tomography versus triple-phase bone scanning. J Bone Joint Surg Br 2005;87:465–70.

37. Scher DM, Pak K, Lonner JH, et al. The predictive value of indium-111 leukocyte scans in the diagnosis of infected total hip, knee, or resection arthroplasties. J Arthroplasty 2000;15:295–300.

38. Zhuang H, Duarte PS, Pourdehnad M, et al. The promising role of 18F-FDG PET in detecting infected lower limb prosthesis implants. J Nucl Med 2001;42: 44–8.

39. Zhuang H, Chacko TK, Hickeson M, et al. Persistent non-specific FDG uptake on PET imaging following hip arthroplasty. Eur J Nucl Med Mol Imaging 2002;29:1328–33.

40. Cheng G. Applications of PET and PET/CT in the evaluation of infection and inflammation in the skeletal system. PET Clinics 2010;5(3):375–85.

41. Manthey N, Reinhard P, Moog F, et al. The use of [18 F]fluorodeoxyglucose positron emission tomography to differentiate between synovitis, loosening and infection of hip and knee prostheses. Nucl Med Commun 2002;23:645–53.

42. Ozuna RM, Delamarter RB. Pyogenic vertebral osteomyelitis and postsurgical disc space infections. Orthop Clin North Am 1996;27:87–94.

43. Mader JT, Shirtliff ME, Bergquist SC, et al. Antimicrobial treatment of chronic osteomyelitis. Clin Orthop Relat Res 1999;(360):47–65.

44. Zimmerli W. Clinical practice. Vertebral osteomyelitis. N Engl J Med 2010;362:1022–9.

45. Mylona E, Samarkos M, Kakalou E, et al. Pyogenic vertebral osteomyelitis: a systematic review of clinical characteristics. Semin Arthritis Rheum 2009;39:10–7.

46. Kowalski TJ, Berbari EF, Huddleston PM, et al. The management and outcome of spinal implant infections: contemporary retrospective cohort study. Clin Infect Dis 2007;44:913–20.

47. Bucher E, Trampuz A, Donati L, et al. Spondylodiscitis associated with bacteraemia due to coagulase-negative staphylococci. Eur J Clin Microbiol Infect Dis 2000;19:118–20.

48. Sobottke R, Zarghooni K, Krengel M, et al. Treatment of spondylodiscitis in human immunodeficiency virus-infected patients: a comparison of conservative

and operative therapy. Spine (Phila Pa 1976) 2009; 34:E452–8.

49. Modic MT, Feiglin DH, Piraino DW, et al. Vertebral osteomyelitis: assessment using MR. Radiology 1985;157:157–66.

50. Tehranzadeh J, Wang F, Mesgarzadeh M. Magnetic resonance imaging of osteomyelitis. Crit Rev Diagn Imaging 1992;33:495–534.

51. Love C, Tomas MB, Tronco GG, et al. FDG PET of infection and inflammation. Radiographics 2005;25: 1357–68.

52. Birmingham MC, Rayner CR, Meagher AK, et al. Linezolid for the treatment of multidrug-resistant, gram-positive infections: experience from a compassionate-use program. Clin Infect Dis 2003;36:159–68.

53. Viola RW, King HA, Adler SM, et al. Delayed infection after elective spinal instrumentation and fusion. A retrospective analysis of eight cases. Spine (Phila Pa 1976) 1997;22:2444–50 [discussion: 2450–1].

54. Love C, Patel M, Lonner BS, et al. Diagnosing spinal osteomyelitis: a comparison of bone and Ga-67 scintigraphy and magnetic resonance imaging. Clin Nucl Med 2000;25:963–77.

55. Liebergall M, Chaimsky G, Lowe J, et al. Pyogenic vertebral osteomyelitis with paralysis. Prognosis and treatment. Clin Orthop Relat Res 1991;(269):142–50.

56. Gratz S, Dorner J, Oestmann JW, et al. 67Ga-citrate and 99Tcm-MDP for estimating the severity of vertebral osteomyelitis. Nucl Med Commun 2000; 21:111–20.

57. de Winter F, van de Wiele C, Vogelaers D, et al. Fluorine-18 fluorodeoxyglucose-position emission tomography: a highly accurate imaging modality for the diagnosis of chronic musculoskeletal infections. J Bone Joint Surg Am 2001;83:651–60.

58. Rothman SL. The diagnosis of infections of the spine by modern imaging techniques. Orthop Clin North Am 1996;27:15–31.

59. Richards BR, Emara KM. Delayed infections after posterior TSRH spinal instrumentation for idiopathic scoliosis: revisited. Spine (Phila Pa 1976) 2001;26:1990–6.

60. Hahn F, Zbinden R, Min K. Late implant infections caused by Propionibacterium acnes in scoliosis surgery. Eur Spine J 2005;14:783–8.

61. Gemmel F, Rijk PC, Collins JM, et al. Expanding role of 18F-fluoro-D-deoxyglucose PET and PET/CT in spinal infections. Eur Spine J 2010;19:540–51.

62. Fang A, Hu SS, Endres N, et al. Risk factors for infection after spinal surgery. Spine (Phila Pa 1976) 2005;30:1460–5.

63. Palestro CJ, Love C. Nuclear medicine and diabetic foot infections. Semin Nucl Med 2009;39:52–65.

64. Sella EJ, Grosser DM. Imaging modalities of the diabetic foot. Clin Podiatr Med Surg 2003;20:729–40.

65. Palestro CJ, Mehta HH, Patel M, et al. Marrow versus infection in the Charcot joint: indium-111 leukocyte and technetium-99m sulfur colloid scintigraphy. J Nucl Med 1998;39:346–50.

66. Nawaz A, Torigian DA, Siegelman ES, et al. Diagnostic performance of FDG-PET, MRI, and plain film radiography (PFR) for the diagnosis of osteomyelitis in the diabetic foot. Mol Imaging Biol 2010;12: 335–42.

67. Hopfner S, Krolak C, Kessler S, et al. Preoperative imaging of Charcot neuroarthropathy in diabetic patients: comparison of ring PET, hybrid PET, and magnetic resonance imaging. Foot Ankle Int 2004; 25:890–5.

68. Kumar R, Basu S, Torigian D, et al. Role of modern imaging techniques for diagnosis of infection in the era of 18F-fluorodeoxyglucose positron emission tomography. Clin Microbiol Rev 2008;21:209–24.

69. Basu S, Chryssikos T, Houseni M, et al. Potential role of FDG PET in the setting of diabetic neuro-osteoarthropathy: can it differentiate uncomplicated Charcot's neuroarthropathy from osteomyelitis and soft-tissue infection? Nucl Med Commun 2007;28: 465–72.

70. Warmann SW, Dittmann H, Seitz G, et al. Follow-up of acute osteomyelitis in children: the possible role of PET/CT in selected cases. J Pediatr Surg 2011; 46:1550–6.

Fever of Unknown Origin: The Roles of FDG PET or PET/CT

Jigang Yang, MD, PhD[a,b], Hongming Zhuang, MD, PhD[c], Sabah Servaes, MD[b,*]

KEYWORDS

- FDG • PET/CT • Fever of unknown origin

Most febrile conditions are readily diagnosed on the basis of presenting symptoms and a problem-focused physical examination. Sometimes, only simple testing, such as a complete blood count or urine culture, is required to make a diagnosis. Viral illnesses (eg, upper respiratory infections) account for most of these self-limiting cases and usually resolve within 2 weeks.[1] When fever persists, it may represent life-threatening or disabling diseases. Persistent fever has associated consequences.[2] For example, febrile seizure is significant in the pediatric population, with an incidence of 5%.[3] High temperature increases cardiac function and oxygen consumption.[4] Fever higher than 41°C can cause brain damage.

CLASSIFICATION OF FEVER OF UNKNOWN ORIGIN IN THE PEDIATRIC POPULATION

Fever of unknown origin (FUO) was defined in 1961 by Petersdorf and Beeson[5] as recurrent fever of 38.3°C or higher, lasting 2 to 3 weeks or longer, and undiagnosed after 1 week of hospital evaluation. The last criterion has undergone modification and is now generally interpreted as no diagnosis after appropriate inpatient or outpatient evaluation.[6] It is now generally accepted that unexplained fever that persists longer than 1 week in a child warrants preliminary investigations, because fever from viral infections generally resolves within that time. Therefore, most recent case series of pediatric FUO included those with pers\istent fever for only 1 or 2 weeks with negative preliminary investigations.[7] Fever is common among pediatric patients. In most clinical settings, the fever is attributable to mild viral infection and is self-limiting[8]; however, persistent fever without known causation in pediatric patients poses a significant challenge to clinicians in terms of patient management. In 2 series of pediatric patients with FUO, it was found that mortality reached more than 5%.[9,10]

Chow and Robinson[7] reviewed data from 1638 patients with FUO and found that infection was by far the most commonly identified etiology of FUO in all studies. In total, the final diagnosis in 51% of patients (832 cases) was infection, with bacterial infections the most common. Fifty-nine percent of patients' infections (491 cases) were caused by bacteria; the most common diagnoses in developed countries were osteomyelitis, tuberculosis, and Bartonellosis and in developing countries were brucellosis, tuberculosis, and typhoid fever. Urinary tract infections are common everywhere. Seven percent (58 cases) of patients' infections were caused by virus, with Epstein-Barr virus accounting for more than half of the cases. Malignancy accounted for 6% of the diagnoses in the analyzed patients (93 cases). The diagnoses of 9% of patients (150 cases) was collagen vascular disease. The diagnoses of 11% of patients (179

[a] Department of Nuclear Medicine, Beijing Friendship Hospital of Capital Medical University, 95 Yong An Road, Xi Cheng District, Beijing 100050, China
[b] Department of Radiology, The Children's Hospital of Philadelphia, University of Pennsylvania School of Medicine, 34th Street and Civic Center Boulevard, Philadelphia, PA 19104, USA
[c] Division of Nuclear Medicine, Department of Radiology, The Children's Hospital of Philadelphia, University of Pennsylvania School of Medicine, 34th Street and Civic Center Boulevard, Philadelphia, PA 19104, USA
* Correspondence author.
E-mail address: servaes@email.chop.edu

PET Clin 7 (2012) 181–189
doi:10.1016/j.cpet.2012.01.006
1556-8598/12/$ – see front matter © 2012 Elsevier Inc. All rights reserved

cases) was categorized as noninfectious etiology with leading diagnoses of Kawasaki disease in developed countries and autoimmune disease and inflammatory bowel disease in developing countries.

IMAGING MODALITIES IN THE EVALUATION OF FUO

Many studies show that identifying the symptoms and clinical history of the patient are a critical component to a successful strategy in the diagnostic workup of FUO. Endoscopy, biopsy, ultrasound, computed tomography (CT), magnetic resonance imaging (MR imaging), and nuclear medicine scintigraphy may be used in some cases. Anatomic imaging modalities, such as ultrasound or CT, should be performed early in the evaluation process to exclude common causes of FUO, such as intra-abdominal abscess or malignancy.[11–13] Ultrasound can detect masses and collections with the benefit of no ionizing radiation; however, its sensitivity is lower than CT.[14,15] MR imaging should generally be used as a second-line modality for clarifying uncertain findings identified by the use of other techniques[11]; however, it is being used more frequently because of its lack of ionizing radiation and the advent of faster MR imaging sequences. In fact, whole-body MR imaging has been advocated in the identification of multifocal disease and has potential in identifying pathology in the patient with FUO.[16] More studies are needed to evaluate the effectiveness of whole-body MR imaging.

Radionuclide imaging allows the detection of focal pathologic changes early in the disease course, even in the absence of a morphologic correlate.[17–20] This sensitivity puts radionuclide imaging at an advantage in comparison with conventional imaging, which depends on detectable anatomic changes. Radiolabeled white blood cells (WBCs) are suited to the evaluation of a focus in occult sepsis.[21] Gallium 67 citrate (67Ga-citrate) can image acute, chronic, granulomatous, and autoimmune inflammation and infection, as well as various malignant diseases. Therefore, 67Ga-citrate was long considered to be the tracer of choice in the evaluation of FUO. The percentage of 67Ga-citrate scans contributing to the final diagnosis was generally found to be higher than that reported for labeled WBCs.[22] Because of the large volume of the patient's blood necessary for the examination, the labeled leukocyte method has only limited utility in small babies.

FDG PET or PET/CT has some advantages over other imaging modalities. It requires less time than gallium or labeled leukocyte scans and the imaging quality and resolution is superior to gallium or labeled leukocyte imaging. FDG is a nonspecific tracer, which is a disadvantage in oncology imaging because of possible false-positive interpretation; the nonspecificity is an advantage in the search of the source of fever of unknown origin because it enables FDG PET to detect both nonmalignant inflammatory and malignant lesions. There is a wide range of accuracy among previous publications regarding how FDG PET/CT can help in finding the source of fever, which is likely related to the patient population involved. In a prospective study involving 74 patients, Buysschaert and colleagues[23] found that FDG PET contributed positively to the diagnosis in 26% of their patients with classical FUO. In another prospective multicenter study involving 70 patients suffering from FUO, Bleeker-Rovers and colleagues[24] found that in 33%, FDG PET was clinically helpful in identifying the source of the fever. It is worth noting that both of these prospective investigations were performed using solely PET, not PET/CT. Studies using PET/CT tend to have much higher accuracy. For example, Keidar and colleagues[25] found that PET/CT identified the underlying cause of fever in 46% of patients with FUO and contributed to the diagnosis or exclusion of a focal pathologic etiology of the febrile state in 90% of patients. A recent study has shown that FDG PET/CT has better accuracy than contrast diagnostic CT in the detection of the source of FUO.[26] It has been proposed that FDG PET might replace other imaging modalities in the evaluation of patients with FUO.[27]

FDG PET OR PET/CT IN THE EVALUATION OF FUO

Infection is the most common cause of FUO in children.[2] Previous studies have shown that FDG PET or PET/CT can detect infection when other diagnostic methods were inconclusive.[28–30] Inflammatory disease ranks the second after infection as a cause of FUO in pediatric patients. Diagnoses responsible for FUO in this population include a large variety of autoimmune and connective tissue diseases, as well as vasculitis syndromes, granulomatous disorders, and endocrine disorders, such as subacute thyroiditis.

Mahfouz and colleagues[31] evaluated the value of FDG PET in the diagnosis of focal infection in patients with multiple myeloma, in which 165 infectious lesions were identified in 143 patients. Many of these infections could not be diagnosed by other methods at the time of their appearance. This study concluded that in patients with multiple myeloma, FDG PET is an effective tool for diagnosing and managing infections. In patients suffering from HIV-associated FUO, FDG PET/CT was helpful for diagnosis in 9 of the 10 patients studied.[32]

Infective endocarditis can also be the source of an FUO. The diagnosis is generally made by echocardiographic identification of valvular vegetations along with clinical assessment; however, vegetations are not always infected. In addition, small vegetations in patients with prosthetic heart valves may escape detection. Yen and colleagues[33] evaluated the effectiveness of FDG PET in the detection of infectious endocarditis. PET images showed FDG uptakes in the corresponding areas detected in echocardiography. They concluded that FDG PET is a promising tool in diagnosing infective endocarditis; however, physiologic cardiac FDG uptake can make this application challenging.

Stumpe and colleagues[34] evaluated the role of FDG PET in detection of soft tissue (**Fig. 1**) and bone infections (39 cases). The sensitivity in soft tissue and bone infection was 96% and 100%, respectively. The specificity is 99% for both. Osteomyelitis is one of the common causes of FUO in the pediatric patient population (**Fig. 2**). Chronic osteomyelitis normally results from inadequately

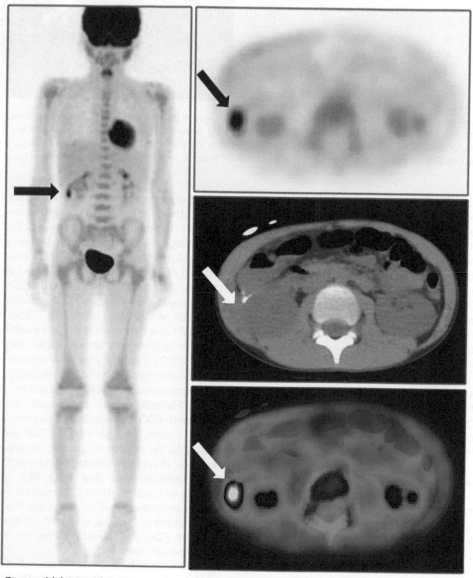

Fig. 1. A 7-year-old boy with a history of relapsed Burkitt lymphoma and FUO. PET images demonstrated increased uptake in the right paracolic gutter (*arrow*). This lesion has a maximum standardized uptake value (SUVmax) of 3.5. The diagnosis of abscess attributable to fistula was later established.

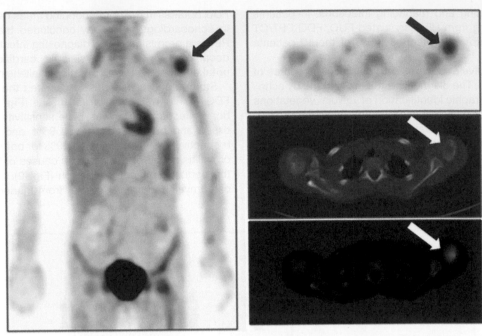

Fig. 2. A 4-year and 9-month-old girl presented with recent severe pain in the left shoulder and fever for more than 1 month. PET images demonstrated diffusely increased bone marrow activity throughout the axial and appendicular skeletons. There is significantly increased FDG activity in the left humeral head (*arrow*), which corresponded to a destructive bony lesion on the low-dose CT images. Osteomyelitis was subsequently established.

treated acute hematogenous osteomyelitis or may follow exogenous bacterial contamination that is attributable to trauma or surgical procedures. In contrast to acute osteomyelitis, chronic osteomyelitis is characterized predominantly by the presence of lymphocyte and plasmocyte infiltrates and a variable amount of necrotic tissue and osteosclerosis.[35] Zhuang and colleagues[36] investigated the value of FDG PET in the diagnosis of possible chronic osteomyelitis and found that the sensitivity, specificity, and accuracy of PET in the evaluation of chronic osteomyelitis was 100.0%, 87.5%, and 91.0%, respectively. Similarly, Guhlmann and colleagues[37] found that the sensitivity and specificity of FDG PET were 100% and 92%, respectively. Other studies of FDG PET in the diagnosis of chronic osteomyelitis have similar conclusions.[38,39] FDG PET study is especially suitable in the evaluation posttraumatic osteomyelitis, because a normal-healing fracture usually has minimal FDG uptake at the fracture site, whereas osteomyelitis will result in intense activity.[40,41] Therefore, FDG PET/CT can effectively distinguish osteomyelitis from normal bone healing following a fracture or surgical intervention.

Vasculitis is another cause of FUO, which is sometimes the presenting symptom.[42] Blockmans and colleagues[43] evaluated the application of FDG PET in patients with vasculitis. Eleven patients and 23 age-matched control volunteers were included in this study. PET imaging showed increased FDG uptake in large thoracic vessels in 4 of 5 cases with polymyalgia rheumatica and in 4 of 6 cases with giant cell arteritis, whereas 1 of 23 control subjects showed FDG uptake (*P*<.001). In Takayasu arteritis, the "pulseless" phase of the disease is generally preceded by nonspecific symptoms. Use of FDG PET in Takayasu arteritis[44–46] and giant cell arteritis[42] has been reported. Giant cell vasculitis, which was temporal artery biopsy–negative but FDG PET/CT–positive, has been reported.[47]

Sarcoidosis is a chronic inflammatory condition of unknown cause, which is another source of FUO. Patients with sarcoidosis may show increased FDG uptake in mediastinal and hilar lymph nodes; the abnormal FDG uptake can extend to the pulmonary parenchyma even in the absence of typical radiologic features.[48,49] It has been demonstrated that FDG PET scan also detects sarcoidosis when 67Ga scan is negative.[50] Brudin and colleagues[51,52] found that the degree of FDG uptake correlates well with disease activity and that FDG PET could be used for monitoring response to treatment.

Subacute thyroiditis, another source of FUO, can easily be diagnosed by typical clinical features, such as neck pain, fever, malaise, myalgia, and fatigue. In atypical cases, FUO may be the only symptom.

18F-FDG PET usually detects painless subacute thyroiditis through a focal or, more commonly, a diffuse increased uptake in the thyroid.[53,54]

FDG PET/CT might play an important role in evaluation of critically ill patients suspected of having an infection. In a study involving 33 patients in the intensive care unit, Simons and colleagues[55] found that PET/CT had a sensitivity of 100% and specificity of 79% in identifying the source of infection.

Because of the ready detection of solid tumors and enlarged lymph nodes by ultrasound, CT, and MR imaging, there is relatively less of a role of FDG PET/CT in diagnosing tumors as the reason for FUO. Tumors are more common in elderly than in pediatric patients with FUO. PET/CT imaging has high sensitivity and specificity in the detection of different malignancies that can cause FUO.[56–62] Not all malignancies demonstrate clear anatomic changes early, and these are times

when PET/CT may be useful. Ozcan and colleagues[63] reported that PET/CT demonstrated acute myeloid leukemia in a patient with FUO.

The experience of FDG PET/CT in the evaluation of FUO in the pediatric population is still limited. Previous research has shown that information acquired from FDG PET is very useful in the management of pediatric liver transplantation candidates suffering with FUO.[64] In an investigation involving a relatively large population of pediatric patients (n = 69) using FDG PET or PET/CT, a diagnosis with FUO or unexplained signs of inflammation could be established in more than half of the patients.[65] The PET or PET/CT scan led to the final diagnoses in 73% of the patients studied.[65]

The data of many previous investigations were largely based solely on PET scanners. Hybrid PET/CT generally yields better results; however, even if PET/CT scanners are used, the CT portion of the study is usually a low-dose, noncontrast,

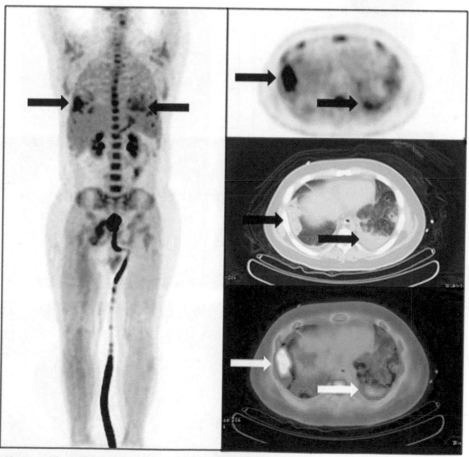

Fig. 3. A 19-year-old male patient with FUO following antibiotic therapy for Klebsiella pneumonia. PET/CT images demonstrated focally increased FDG uptake bilaterally in the lower lungs (*arrows*), which correlated to infiltrates on the low-dose CT images. There were bilateral pleural effusions with mild FDG uptake. There were multiple foci of consolidation within the bilateral lungs with mild FDG uptake. The findings were also shown on anatomic imaging and are consistent with multifocal pneumonia.

nondiagnostic study. Use of FDG PET/high-resolution diagnostic contrast CT in FUO evaluation might be able to increase the sensitivity of the study. Balink and colleagues[66] used this approach to evaluate FUO and successfully identified the source of fever in more than half of the 41 patients assessed. The results from Ferda and colleagues,[67] who also used this approach, are even more promising. In this study, the authors evaluated 48 patients with FUO and the source of the fever was correctly identified in 43 patients; however, such practice renders a much higher radiation dose to the patient. Therefore, this method should not be generalized before more data can emerge to justify such practice.

Some investigators believe that FDG PET is useful only in adult patients with FUO who have elevated erythrocyte sedimentation rate (ESR) and C-reactive protein (CRP) but is less likely to be helpful in patients with normal ESR and CRP.[24] In a separate investigation involving a similar number of adult patients with FUO, however, others concluded that ESR and CRP could not predict the usefulness of FDG PET.[23] In the pediatric population, the only published large-scale study also indicated that laboratory and clinical parameters of the children did not predict the usefulness of FDG PET scans.[65] Further study is necessary to assess whether the levels of ESR or CRP can play a role in predicting the usefulness of PET/CT in the evaluation of patients with FUO.

Early use of FDG PET/CT in the evaluation of patients with FUO can be cost saving. Although it is debatable exactly what percentage of the source of FUO can be detected by FDG PET/CT, it is generally agreeable that the FDG PET/CT

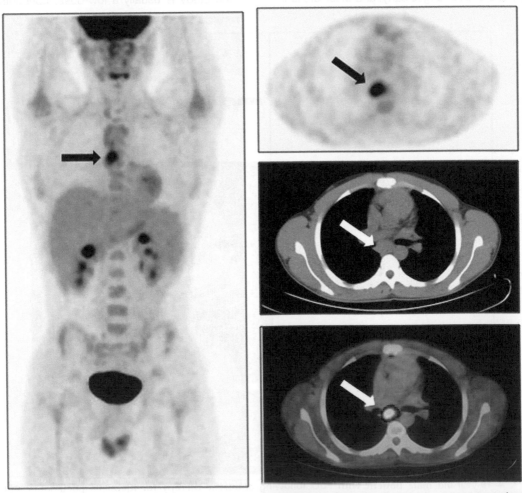

Fig. 4. A 16-year-old boy with FUO. Abnormality was not appreciated on the diagnostic, noncontrast chest CT images, which were performed 9 days before PET/CT. PET images demonstrate a focus of intense FDG uptake (SUVmax of 6.5) in the mediastinum (*arrow*), corresponding to a 23 × 16-mm subcarinal lymph node on the low-dose CT images. Pathology demonstrated histiocytosis and hemophagocytosis.

has a very high negative predictive value up to 100% in excluding focal lesions.[66] Keidar and colleagues[25] reported that in all 21 patients with FUO who had negative PET/CT results, a localized lesion was never found in a clinical follow-up period of more than 12 months. In general, there is always a positive FDG PET/CT finding if there is a positive anatomic imaging result (Fig. 3). Conversely, a positive FDG PET finding is not always preceded with a positive anatomic imaging result (Fig. 4). It is conceivable that the most effective strategy when there is a negative FDG PET/CT, is not to perform any further imaging by other modalities. In support of this plan is the finding that in patients in the intensive care unit who are suspected of infection, a normal FDG PET/CT excludes important infections requiring prolonged antibiotic therapy or drainage.[55] By identifying the source of the fever or excluding focal lesions earlier, FDG PET/CT is able to reduce unnecessary tests and shorten hospitalization days. Therefore, FDG PET/CT use may be cost-effective, especially if performed in an early stage of FUO evaluation.[68]

SUMMARY

FDG PET/CT study is cost-effective in the evaluation of FUO if used at an early stage, by helping to establish an early diagnosis and reducing hospitalization days owing to diagnostic purposes and the performance of unnecessary tests.[68] When systemic diseases are excluded, FDG PET/CT has a negative predictive value of 100%.[25,66] If FDG PET/CT failed to identify the source of the fever, the cause of the fever is unlikely to be found by any other modality. In addition, when PET/CT results are negative, it is unlikely the patient's fever will progress.[29] A PET/CT scan is ideally performed early in the diagnostic workup of patients with FUO.[28,29]

REFERENCES

1. Dykewicz MS. 7. Rhinitis and sinusitis. J Allergy Clin Immunol 2003;111:S520–9.
2. Akpede GO, Akenzua GI. Aetiology and management of children with acute fever of unknown origin. Paediatr Drugs 2001;3:169–93.
3. Maytal J, Shinnar S. Febrile status epilepticus. Pediatrics 1990;86:611–6.
4. Drwal-Klein LA, Phelps SJ. Antipyretic therapy in the febrile child. Clin Pharm 1992;11:1005–21.
5. Petersdorf RG, Beeson PB. Fever of unexplained origin: report on 100 cases. Medicine (Baltimore) 1961;40:1–30.
6. Petersdorf RG. Fever of unknown origin. An old friend revisited. Arch Intern Med 1992;152:21–2.
7. Chow A, Robinson JL. Fever of unknown origin in children: a systematic review. World J Pediatr 2011;7:5–10.
8. Finkelstein JA, Christiansen CL, Platt R. Fever in pediatric primary care: occurrence, management, and outcomes. Pediatrics 2000;105:260–6.
9. Lohr JA, Hendley JO. Prolonged fever of unknown origin: a record of experiences with 54 childhood patients. Clin Pediatr (Phila) 1977;16:768–73.
10. Pizzo PA, Lovejoy FH Jr, Smith DH. Prolonged fever in children: review of 100 cases. Pediatrics 1975;55:468–73.
11. Mourad O, Palda V, Detsky AS. A comprehensive evidence-based approach to fever of unknown origin. Arch Intern Med 2003;163:545–51.
12. Gayer G, Ben Ely A, Maymon R, et al. Enlargement of the spleen as an incidental finding on CT in post-partum females with fever. Br J Radiol 2011. [Epub ahead of print].
13. Addley HC, Green L, Petitclerc S. Acute dengue fever with computed tomography (CT) correlation. Am J Trop Med Hyg 2011;84:651–2.
14. Jasinski RW, Glazer GM, Francis IR, et al. CT and ultrasound in abscess detection at specific anatomic sites: a study of 198 patients. Comput Radiol 1987;11:41–7.
15. El Khoury AC, Durden E, Ma L, et al. Perception and management of fever in infants up to six months of age: a survey of US pediatricans. BMC Pediatr 2010;10:95.
16. Kellenberger CJ, Epelman M, Miller SF, et al. Fast STIR whole-body MR imaging in children. Radiographics 2004;24:1317–30.
17. Dadparvar S, Anderson GS, Bhargava P, et al. Paraneoplastic encephalitis associated with cystic teratoma is detected by fluorodeoxyglucose positron emission tomography with negative magnetic resonance image findings. Clin Nucl Med 2003;28:893–6.
18. Codreanu I, Zhuang H. Isolated cholangiolitis revealed by 18F-FDG-PET/CT in a patient with fever of unknown origin. Hell J Nucl Med 2011;14:60–1.
19. Chamroonrat W, Cheng G, Servaes S, et al. Cytomegalovirus pneumonitis detected by gallium-67 scintigraphy with a negative diagnostic chest computed tomography. Clin Nucl Med 2010;35:542–4.
20. Makis W, Abikhzer G, Stern J. Incidental early stage endometrial adenocarcinoma diagnosed by F-18 FDG PET-CT, which was negative on ultrasound and nonspecific on MRI. Clin Nucl Med 2010;35:265–6.
21. Meller J, Becker W. [Nuclear medicine diagnosis of patients with fever of unknown origin (FUO)]. Nuklearmedizin 2001;40:59–70 [in German].
22. Knockaert DC, Mortelmans LA, De Roo MC, et al. Clinical value of gallium-67 scintigraphy in evaluation of fever of unknown origin. Clin Infect Dis 1994;18:601–5.

23. Buysschaert I, Vanderschueren S, Blockmans D, et al. Contribution of (18)fluoro-deoxyglucose positron emission tomography to the work-up of patients with fever of unknown origin. Eur J Intern Med 2004; 15:151–6.

24. Bleeker-Rovers CP, Vos FJ, Mudde AH, et al. A prospective multi-centre study of the value of FDG-PET as part of a structured diagnostic protocol in patients with fever of unknown origin. Eur J Nucl Med Mol Imaging 2007;34:694–703.

25. Keidar Z, Gurman-Balbir A, Gaitini D, et al. Fever of unknown origin: the role of 18F-FDG PET/CT. J Nucl Med 2008;49:1980–5.

26. Rosenbaum J, Basu S, Beckerman S, et al. Evaluation of diagnostic performance of (18)F-FDG-PET compared to CT in detecting potential causes of fever of unknown origin in an academic centre. Hell J Nucl Med 2011;14:255–9.

27. Meller J, Sahlmann CO, Scheel AK. 18F-FDG PET and PET/CT in fever of unknown origin. J Nucl Med 2007;48:35–45.

28. Pedersen TI, Roed C, Knudsen LS, et al. Fever of unknown origin: a retrospective study of 52 cases with evaluation of the diagnostic utility of FDG-PET/CT. Scand J Infect Dis 2012;44(1):18–23.

29. Pelosi E, Skanjeti A, Penna D, et al. Role of integrated PET/CT with [(18)F]-FDG in the management of patients with fever of unknown origin: a single-centre experience. Radiol Med 2011;116:809–20.

30. Kubota K, Nakamoto Y, Tamaki N, et al. FDG-PET for the diagnosis of fever of unknown origin: a Japanese multi-center study. Ann Nucl Med 2011;25:355–64.

31. Mahfouz T, Miceli MH, Saghafifar F, et al. 18F-fluoro-deoxyglucose positron emission tomography contributes to the diagnosis and management of infections in patients with multiple myeloma: a study of 165 infectious episodes. J Clin Oncol 2005;23: 7857–63.

32. Castaigne C, Tondeur M, de Wit S, et al. Clinical value of FDG-PET/CT for the diagnosis of human immunodeficiency virus-associated fever of unknown origin: a retrospective study. Nucl Med Commun 2009;30:41–7.

33. Yen RF, Chen YC, Wu YW, et al. Using 18-fluoro-2-deoxyglucose positron emission tomography in detecting infectious endocarditis/endoarteritis: a preliminary report. Acad Radiol 2004;11:316–21.

34. Stumpe KD, Dazzi H, Schaffner A, et al. Infection imaging using whole-body FDG-PET. Eur J Nucl Med 2000;27:822–32.

35. Mader JT, Shirtliff M, Calhoun JH. Staging and staging application in osteomyelitis. Clin Infect Dis 1997;25.1303–9.

36. Zhuang H, Duarte PS, Pourdehand M, et al. Exclusion of chronic osteomyelitis with F-18 fluorodeoxyglucose positron emission tomographic imaging. Clin Nucl Med 2000;25:281–4.

37. Guhlmann A, Brecht-Krauss D, Suger G, et al. Chronic osteomyelitis: detection with FDG PET and correlation with histopathologic findings. Radiology 1998;206:749–54.

38. Hakim SG, Bruecker CW, Jacobsen H, et al. The value of FDG-PET and bone scintigraphy with SPECT in the primary diagnosis and follow-up of patients with chronic osteomyelitis of the mandible. Int J Oral Maxillofac Surg 2006;35:809–16.

39. Hartmann A, Eid K, Dora C, et al. Diagnostic value of 18F-FDG PET/CT in trauma patients with suspected chronic osteomyelitis. Eur J Nucl Med Mol Imaging 2007;34:704–14.

40. Zhuang H, Sam JW, Chacko TK, et al. Rapid normalization of osseous FDG uptake following traumatic or surgical fractures. Eur J Nucl Med Mol Imaging 2003;30:1096–103.

41. Koort JK, Makinen TJ, Knuuti J, et al. Comparative 18F-FDG PET of experimental Staphylococcus aureus osteomyelitis and normal bone healing. J Nucl Med 2004;45:1406–11.

42. Czihal M, Tato F, Forster S, et al. Fever of unknown origin as initial manifestation of large vessel giant cell arteritis: diagnosis by colour-coded sonography and 18-FDG-PET. Clin Exp Rheumatol 2010;28:549–52.

43. Blockmans D, Maes A, Stroobants S, et al. New arguments for a vasculitic nature of polymyalgia rheumatica using positron emission tomography. Rheumatology (Oxford) 1999;38:444–7.

44. Shih G, Shih WJ, Huang WS, et al. Hashimoto thyroiditis and Takayasu aortitis: visualization of the thyroid gland and ring appearance of the mediastinum on F-18-FDG PET. Clin Nucl Med 2008;33: 377–9.

45. Lee SG, Ryu JS, Kim HO, et al. Evaluation of disease activity using F-18 FDG PET-CT in patients with Takayasu arteritis. Clin Nucl Med 2009;34:749–52.

46. Miyachi H, Kodani E, Okazaki R, et al. [A case of fever of unknown origin that diagnosed as early-phase of Takayasu arteritis by FDG-PET/CT]. Nippon Naika Gakkai Zasshi 2011;100:1388–90 [in Japanese].

47. Schafer VS, Warrington KJ, Williamson EE, et al. Delayed diagnosis of biopsy-negative giant cell arteritis presenting as fever of unknown origin. J Gen Intern Med 2009;24:532–6.

48. Keijsers RG, Grutters JC, Thomeer M, et al. Imaging the inflammatory activity of sarcoidosis: sensitivity and inter observer agreement of 67Ga imaging and 18F-FDG PET. Q J Nucl Med Mol Imaging 2011;55:66–71.

49. Basu S, Asopa RV, Baghel NS. Early documentation of therapeutic response at 6 weeks following corticosteroid therapy in extensive sarcoidosis: promise of FDG-PET. Clin Nucl Med 2009;34:689–90.

50. Xiu Y, Yu JQ, Cheng E, et al. Sarcoidosis demonstrated by FDG PET imaging with negative findings on gallium scintigraphy. Clin Nucl Med 2005;30:193–5.

51. Brudin LH, Valind SO, Rhodes CG, et al. Fluorine-18 deoxyglucose uptake in sarcoidosis measured with positron emission tomography. Eur J Nucl Med 1994;21:297–305.

52. Zhuang H, Alavi A. 18-Fluorodeoxyglucose positron emission tomographic imaging in the detection and monitoring of infection and inflammation. Semin Nucl Med 2002;32:47–59.

53. Lambert M, Jouret F, Lonneux M, et al. Mismatch of F-18 fluorodeoxyglucose (FDG) positron emission tomography (PET) and Tc-99m pertechnetate thyroid scan in subacute thyroiditis. Acta Clin Belg 2008;63:209–10.

54. Song YS, Jang SJ, Chung JK, et al. F-18 fluorodeoxyglucose (FDG) positron emission tomography (PET) and Tc-99m pertechnate scan findings of a patient with unilateral subacute thyroiditis. Clin Nucl Med 2009;34:456–8.

55. Simons KS, Pickkers P, Bleeker-Rovers CP, et al. F-18-fluorodeoxyglucose positron emission tomography combined with CT in critically ill patients with suspected infection. Intensive Care Med 2010;36:504–11.

56. Rhodes MM, Delbeke D, Whitlock JA, et al. Utility of FDG-PET/CT in follow-up of children treated for Hodgkin and non-Hodgkin lymphoma. J Pediatr Hematol Oncol 2006;28:300–6.

57. Amthauer H, Furth C, Denecke T, et al. FDG-PET in 10 children with non-Hodgkin's lymphoma: initial experience in staging and follow-up. Klin Padiatr 2005;217:327–33.

58. Lee MK, Kwon CG, Hwang KH, et al. F-18 FDG PET/CT findings in a case of undifferentiated embryonal sarcoma of the liver with lung and adrenal gland metastasis in a child. Clin Nucl Med 2009;34:107–8.

59. Ak I, Stokkel MP, Pauwels EK. Positron emission tomography with 2-[18F]fluoro-2-deoxy-D-glucose in oncology. Part II. The clinical value in detecting and staging primary tumours. J Cancer Res Clin Oncol 2000;126:560–74.

60. Partridge S, Timothy A, O'Doherty MJ, et al. 2-Fluorine-18-fluoro-2-deoxy-D glucose positron emission tomography in the pretreatment staging of Hodgkin's disease: influence on patient management in a single institution. Ann Oncol 2000;11:1273–9.

61. Munker R, Glass J, Griffeth LK, et al. Contribution of PET imaging to the initial staging and prognosis of patients with Hodgkin's disease. Ann Oncol 2004; 15:1699–704.

62. Rigacci L, Vitolo U, Nassi L, et al. Positron emission tomography in the staging of patients with Hodgkin's lymphoma. A prospective multicentric study by the Intergruppo Italiano Linfomi. Ann Hematol 2007;86: 897–903.

63. Ozcan K P, Kara Gedik G, Sari O, et al. Acute myeloid leukemia detected on fluorine-18 fluorodeoxyglucose positron emission tomography/computed tomography imaging in a patient with fever of unknown origin. Rev Esp Med Nucl 2011; 30:115–6.

64. Sturm E, Rings EH, Scholvinck EH, et al. Fluorodeoxyglucose positron emission tomography contributes to management of pediatric liver transplantation candidates with fever of unknown origin. Liver Transpl 2006;12:1698–704.

65. Jasper N, Dabritz J, Frosch M, et al. Diagnostic value of [(18)F]-FDG PET/CT in children with fever of unknown origin or unexplained signs of inflammation. Eur J Nucl Med Mol Imaging 2010;37: 136–45.

66. Balink H, Collins J, Bruyn GA, et al. F-18 FDG PET/CT in the diagnosis of fever of unknown origin. Clin Nucl Med 2009;34:862–8.

67. Ferda J, Ferdova E, Zahlava J, et al. Fever of unknown origin: a value of (18)F-FDG-PET/CT with integrated full diagnostic isotropic CT imaging. Eur J Radiol 2010;73:518–25.

68. Becerra Nakayo EM, Garcia Vicente AM, Soriano Castrejon AM, et al. Analysis of cost-effectiveness in the diagnosis of fever of unknown origin and the role of (18)F-FDG PET-CT: a proposal of diagnostic algorithm. Rev Esp Med Nucl 2011. [Epub ahead of print].

PET/CT in Patients with Sarcoidosis or IgG4 Disease

Jian Q. Yu, MD, FRCPC[a],*, Mohan Doss, PhD, MCCPM[a],
Ion Codreanu, MD, PhD[b], Hongming Zhuang, MD, PhD[b]

KEYWORDS

- PET • PET/CT • FDG • Sarcoidosis • Inflammation
- Infection

Sarcoidosis is a disorder of unknown origin that affects individuals at different geographic locations and is characterized by the presence of multisystem noncaseating granulomas. It was first described by a dermatologist, Dr Jonathan Hutchinson in 1877,[1] who reported his findings in a 50-year-old man who had large purple skin plaques on his hands and feet and in a 64-year-old woman with large purple patches on her face and arms. Since this initial description, histopatho-histologic characteristics of this disorder have been clearly defined and are the bases for making the diagnosis. This disease affects young adults more often than those who are older, and generally presents with pulmonary manifestations, but other organs/systems, including the skin, eyes, muscles, heart, and brain, can be affected initially or at later stages of the disease.

The exact prevalence of sarcoidosis is still unknown. Its incidence is different at various geographic locations around the world and in the United States, and it is more commonly noted in African American populations than in other ethnic groups. It has been estimated that the lifetime risk of sarcoidosis in blacks in the United States is 2.4%, compared with a lifetime risk of 0.85% in whites.[2]

The origin and pathogenesis of sarcoidosis are still unclear. Sarcoidosis is generally hypothesized to multiple causes, which can explain the different patterns and manifestations of the illness.[3] Assessment of disease using conventional imaging methods is difficult and unreliable. However, accurate determination of disease activity is essential for timely administration of corticosteroids to control the disease and relieve the symptoms. The natural course of the disease in individual patients is variable. Although sarcoidosis is self-limiting in many patients, approximately 10% develop serious disability from the disease, with a mortality rate of 5%. This article focuses on the role of imaging modalities for the initial and follow-up assessment of sarcoidosis.

DIAGNOSTIC IMAGING STUDIES

More than 90% of sarcoidosis is detected through the abnormalities noted on conventional chest radiograph or CT images of the thorax. In many cases, the conclusion is reached through exclusion of other pathologies. Bilateral hilar adenopathy is the classic chest radiograph finding indicative of sarcoidosis, but it is not specific for sarcoidosis. Parenchymal infiltrates seen in a segment of the population may be interstitial, alveolar, or both. Infrequently (for <5% of patients) pleural involvement can result in lymphocytic exudative effusion, chylothorax, hemothorax, or pneumothorax. Invasive procedures, such as biopsies guided by CT or ultrasound, mediastinoscopy, open lung biopsy, bronchoscopy, or other endoscopic techniques, are not discussed in this

[a] Nuclear Medicine/PET Service, Department of Diagnostic Imaging, Fox Chase Cancer Center, 333 Cottman Avenue, Philadelphia, PA 19111, USA
[b] Division of Nuclear Medicine, Department of Radiology, The Children's Hospital of Philadelphia, University of Pennsylvania School of Medicine, 34th Street and Civic Center Boulevard, Philadelphia, PA 19104, USA
* Corresponding author.
E-mail address: Michael.Yu@fccc.edu

PET Clin 7 (2012) 191–210
doi:10.1016/j.cpet.2012.01.005
1556-8598/12/$ – see front matter © 2012 Elsevier Inc. All rights reserved.

article, but are valuable in obtaining specimens for final diagnosis.

Chest Radiograph

The classification of pulmonary involvement in sarcoidosis is based on the radiographic stage of the disease:

Stage I: bilateral hilar adenopathy only. Fifty percent of affected patients exhibit bilateral hilar adenopathy as the first expression of sarcoidosis.

Stage II: bilateral hilar adenopathy and interstitial infiltrates (the latter occurs more often in the upper rather than in the lower lung zones). These findings are present at the initial diagnosis in 25% of patients.

Stage III: interstitial disease with shrinking hilar nodes. Interstitial opacities are commonly present at this stage and are predominantly distributed in the upper lung zones.

Stage IV: advanced bilateral fibrosis of the lungs.

Additional pulmonary findings that can occur in patients with sarcoidosis include:

- Nodular opacities
- Endobronchial involvement in 40% of patients with stage I and in 70% of patients with stages II and III disease
- Significant stenosis of the airways; this abnormality is uncommon and can cause significant morbidity when it is severe
- Submucosal noncaseating epithelioid granulomas of the lower and upper airways, including the larynx, pharynx, and sinuses.

Although the chest radiograph provides a useful anatomic guide for assessing lung involvement, it cannot determine disease activity and functional consequences of the inflammatory process in the affected sites. In general, chest radiograph findings are noted late in the course of the disease, and monitoring response to treatment is limited using this imaging technique.

CT Scan

Tomographic images show a variety of abnormalities and overall are more accurate and sensitive than chest radiographs in assessing the presence and extent of the disease. The CT findings can be one or more of the following:

- Hilar and mediastinal lymphadenopathy
- Beaded or irregular thickening of the bronchovascular bundles
- Nodules along bronchi, vessels, and subpleural regions
- Bronchial wall thickening

- Ground glass opacification
- Parenchymal masses or consolidation
- Parenchymal bands
- Cysts
- Traction bronchiectasis
- Fibrosis with distortion of the lung architecture.

High-resolution CT (HRCT) scanning shows the predominance of these changes in the mid-to-upper zone. It can also detect parenchymal abnormalities that are not seen in the plain chest radiograph.

The HRCT findings correlate well with the histologic abnormalities. Ground-glass opacities, for example, are associated with sarcoid granulomas rather than alveolitis. This finding has raised the question of whether alveolitis is a prominent feature of sarcoidosis. Alveolitis is rarely identified in patients with clinically significant disease. CT scan is useful for detecting recurrence, but the sensitivity of the technique is suboptimal for detecting early disease.

MRI

MRI is useful for suspected neurosarcoidosis and other solid organ involvement, but its role in assessing pulmonary sarcoidosis is still limited. MRI is also of value in detecting cardiac involvement of sarcoidosis because of advancements in equipment and acquisition techniques.

Conventional Nuclear Medicine Methods

Gallium-67 scintigraphy

Gallium-67 scintigraphy is one of the earliest techniques used for diagnosis and management of sarcoidosis. This radiotracer localizes at the inflammatory sites in the lung but not in the normal parenchyma. Whole-body gallium scanning has been used as a sensitive but nonspecific indicator of disease activity in other organs. It is particularly useful for diagnosing the disease in patients with normal chest radiographs and or otherwise atypical presentations. Patterns of symmetrically increased uptake in the mediastinal and hilar nodes (lambda sign) and in the lacrimal, parotid, and salivary glands (panda sign) are considered pathognomonic for sarcoidosis and are well known to nuclear medicine physicians and sarcoidosis experts.[4] Gallium scanning may guide clinicians to the appropriate biopsy sites and may help determine whether radiologic densities represent reversible inflammation or fibrosis. Gallium uptake is affected by systemic administration of corticosteroids, and thus a negative scan in patients being treated with prednisone may be unreliable for detecting active disease. However, a negative study may indicate a favorable response to this drug.

A direct relationship has been shown between a visual index of gallium-67 uptake in the lung and the number of inflammatory cells (particularly macrophages) recovered through bronchoalveolar lavage in patients with sarcoidosis (and idiopathic pulmonary fibrosis). Therefore, the degree of uptake of gallium-67 may be useful in determining the level of alveolar inflammation in these patients, because the agent is primarily concentrated in the alveolar macrophages and, to a lesser degree, in the neutrophils. In addition, studies in normal subjects have shown that a small but significant amount of gallium-67 in the alveolar macrophages obtained through bronchoalveolar lavage is detected despite negative pulmonary images.

Gallium-67 lung scanning is not recommended for the routine evaluation of patients with suspected or known sarcoidosis. In general, the study is difficult to interpret, the findings are nonspecific, and a negative scan does not exclude disease. However, it can be used in clinical settings in which state-of-the-art imaging studies (such as PET) are not available or are inconclusive.[5] Gallium-67 scanning also has been accepted as a tool for monitoring response to therapy for patients with positive baseline examinations. Whole-body gallium-67 study is useful for identifying clinically silent sites in which to obtain tissue for biopsy to aid in diagnosis.

Thallium-201 and technetium 99m sestamibi

Thallium-201 and technetium (Tc) 99m sestamibi imaging have been used as techniques to diagnose cardiac sarcoid, differentiate it from coronary artery disease, and monitor response to treatment. These imaging modalities are discussed in more detail elsewhere in the cardiac sarcoidosis section of this article.

Other radiotracers

Recently, some newer radiotracers have been used for the diagnosis and assessment of patients with sarcoidosis, such as depreotide and other somatostatin receptor imaging agents. A prospective pilot study using Tc 99m–labeled depreotide in 22 patients with known sarcoidosis showed that this agent binds to specific somatostatin receptors.[6] Scans were positive in 18 patients (81%), and all four patients with negative scans had normal plain chest radiographs. In addition, the study showed all sites of nonpulmonary lesions. The images correlated well with the disease stage as determined with chest radiographs and pulmonary function tests. However, this compound is no longer available from commercial vendors for clinical or research use in the United States.

In another study, results of gallium-67 scans and indium-111–labeled pentetreotide were compared in patients with sarcoidosis.[7] The latter tracer is a peptide that binds to the somatostatin receptors. Results showed the superiority of peptide imaging over gallium-67 scanning not only on a patient-by-patient basis (18/18 positive scans for peptide vs 16/18 positive results for gallium-67) but also on a lesion-by-lesion basis (64/99 lesions positive for gallium-67 vs 82/99 positive for peptide). This head-to-head comparison shows that somatostatin receptor imaging may prove to be superior to gallium-67 scan in the management of these patients.

PET

The remainder of this article is devoted to the role of PET imaging in assessing patients with sarcoidosis.

Role of 18F-fluorodeoxyglucose PET for Assessing Sarcoidosis

PET with 18F-fluorodeoxyglucose (FDG) is being increasingly used to examine patients with cancer and those with cardiac and neurologic disorders. Until recently, the standard PET scans consisted of the emission scan followed by the acquisition of radionuclide transmission scan for the purpose of attenuation correction, with the complete scan taking 1 hour or more to complete. Currently, hybrid PET/CT scanners that combine the functional PET with anatomic information from CT have become common, with the improvement in the technologies reducing the duration of complete scans to typically less than a half-hour. The CT scan is not only used for localization but also for attenuation correction. In the United States, PET/CT has become the norm, with most PET studies being conducted with integrated PET/CT scanners.

Recently, the role of FDG PET imaging in the evaluation of inflammatory and infectious processes has been widely explored.[8–16] Sarcoidosis as an inflammatory disorder is an appropriate candidate for this powerful technique. The typical appearance of the sarcoidosis is activity in the hilum bilaterally and the mediastinum (Fig. 1).

The modern PET/CT study has several advantages. One is the large area of the body covered in a routine scan: from base of skull to the upper/mid thigh. Sarcoidosis is often a multiple-organ disease, and because the common PET/CT scans cover more area of the body than other imaging modalities, they can evaluate the extent of the

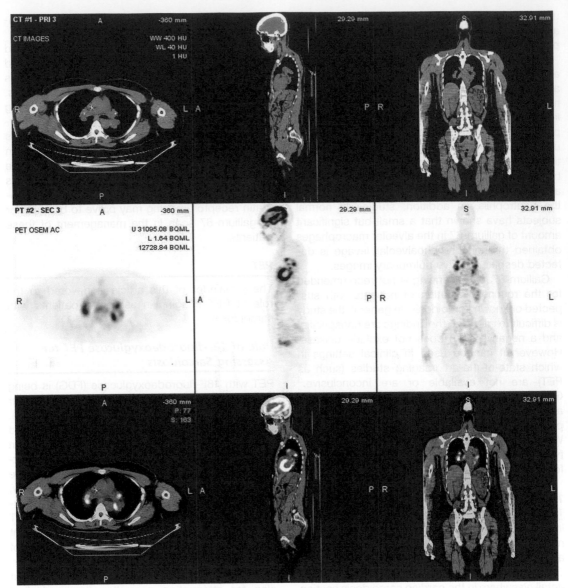

Fig. 1. Posttherapy PET/CT scan of a 57-year-old white woman with history of colorectal cancer. No significant abnormal activity is seen in the gastrointestinal tract or the liver. However, multiple foci of increased activity are seen in both hilar regions and throughout the mediastinum. The patient has a known history of sarcoidosis, and the observed distribution is the typical pattern in the thorax for sarcoidosis. The top row is CT images; the middle row is PET images, and the lower row is PET and CT fused display. The projections shown are in transaxial, sagittal, and coronal slices from left to right.

disease more thoroughly.[17–20] A recent study by Teirstein and colleagues[21] with 188 scans in 137 patients with sarcoidosis found that PET scans are of value in identifying occult and reversible granulomas. The other advantage of PET/CT is that calcification in the lymph nodes from the inflammatory diseases such as sarcoid can be detected easily with the CT portion of the PET/CT procedure (**Fig. 2**).

PULMONARY SARCOIDOSIS

The first report of FDG PET imaging in sarcoidosis appeared in the literature in late 1980s in meeting abstracts. The first published report of FDG PET for differential diagnosis of sarcoidosis was a case report in 1994 involving two patients.[22] Two editorials in the same issue of the journal projected a role for this methodology in the management of patients with this disorder.[8,23] These

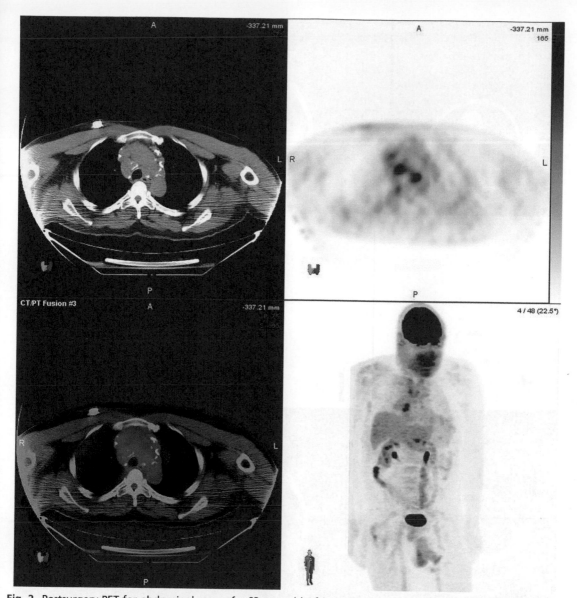

Fig. 2. Postsurgery PET for abdominal mass of a 62-year-old African American man. Linear activity is seen in the abdomen consistent with postprocedure inflammation. Focal activity is noted in the mediastinal nodes with calcifications. After further review, a family history of sarcoid was noted. The patient was free from metastatic disease in follow-up scans. The top row is transaxial CT and PET images from left to right. The bottom row is fused PET/CT images and maximum-intensity projection display of the whole-body PET.

articles indicated that PET may not be a major tool for the initial diagnosis of sarcoidosis, but it may play a role in the management of patients with this disorder. Since then, several case reports have been published in the literature describing patients who were discovered to have sarcoid incidentally with FDG PET imaging.[22,24–26] In one case, recurrent sarcoidosis was discovered in transplanted lungs.[27] Incidentally detected sarcoidosis has been interpreted as cancer in the settings of a workup for malignant disease.[28–30]

Because of increased reports in the literature, most experienced imaging experts will include sarcoid in the differential diagnosis when the FDG distribution shows the typical pattern. In clinical practice, pathology leads to the final diagnosis. This article presents a case in Fox Chase Cancer Center: a patient with typical pattern of sarcoid distribution. However, because of a patient history of smoking, lung nodules, and high suspicion of malignancy, an invasive procedure was performed to obtain tissue diagnosis (**Fig. 3**). As

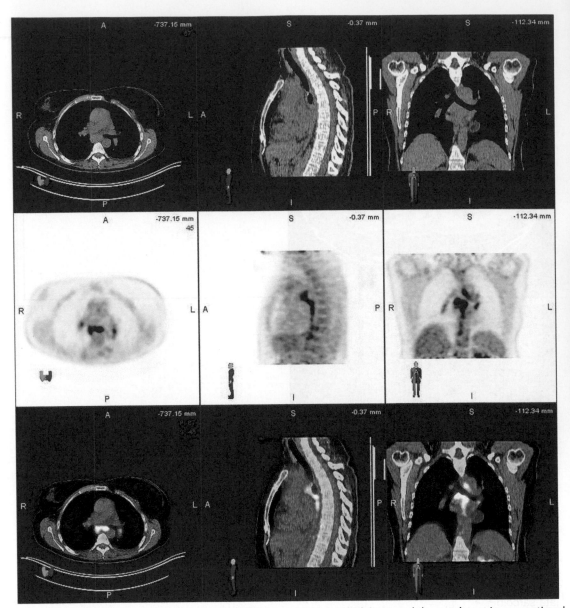

Fig. 3. Delayed PET/CT images of the thorax of a 45-year-old smoker with lung nodules are shown in conventional display. The top row is CT images, the middle row is PET images, and the lower row is PET and CT fused display. All images are in transaxial, sagittal, and coronal slice from left to right. The activity in the nodules are not elevated (not shown). The activity in the mediastinum and hilum is typical of the pattern for sarcoid or inflammatory disease. Because of a high suspicion of malignancy, tissue was obtained from mediastinoscopy with no tumor found and sarcoidosis confirmed.

for oncologists, tissue biopsy is always an important and essential part of the diagnosis.[31–35]

A case report has shown the superiority of FDG PET scan over gallium-67 scan for diagnosing this disease.[36] In this patient, the FDG PET images showed extensive disease activity in the chest and brain, whereas gallium 67 study was unremarkable. Another study has examined 28 patients at various stages of the disease with

FDG PET scans.[14] All patients had either established diagnosis or CT findings that were suggestive of sarcoidosis. The typical patterns on FDG PET images were similar to those in the gallium-67 images and included bilateral hilar activity extending to the mediastinum and lung parenchyma. This pattern was seen in 71% of the FDG PET images in this study. The second observation was a significant discrepancy between PET and

CT scans in 19% of the cases, with the PET scan showing multiple foci of intense activity both within and outside the chest, whereas CT showed only a solitary nodule. Activity in the spleen was seen commonly in this group of patients. Response to treatment was more clearly detected with PET than with CT imaging. Because CT scan is sensitive for detecting focal malignant lesions in findings (positive PET and negative CT) in the lungs, discrepancy between PET and CT scans should be considered as indicative of the possibility of sarcoidosis. In 10% of this group, CT scans showed multiple small lesions in the lungs that were suggestive of metastases from an unknown primary tumor. FDG PET showed a similar finding in the lungs and but no metastases elsewhere in the body. This discrepancy indicated the possibility of an inflammatory process in the lungs, such as sarcoidosis, which was later proven correct by further studies.

A more recent article by Nishiyama and coworkers[37] did a comparative evaluation of FDG PET and gallium-67 scintigraphy in patients with sarcoidosis. They used both visual assessment and semi-quantitative analysis: standardized uptake value (SUV) for PET and ratio of lesion to normal lumbar spine (L/N ratio) for gallium scan. The SUV usually highlights the disease much more than the L/N ratio. The investigators' conclusion is not surprising: FDG PET can detect pulmonary lesions as well as gallium-67 scintigraphy. However, FDG PET seems to be more accurate and contributes to a better evaluation of extrapulmonary disease in patients with sarcoidosis. Other articles are in agreement.[38,39] The latest article by a Netherlands group[40] concluded that PET is more sensitive than gallium-67 scan, is better for detection of extrapulmonary lesions, and has good interobserver agreement. They suggest PET scans as a preferred method to evaluate sarcoidosis.

Sarcoidosis can be diagnosed based on the typical/classical patterns of the uptake of either FDG or other tracers.[22,28,41–43] However, it can frequently mimic malignant disorders and therefore is a source of false-positive findings, as noted in published literature.[24,44–55] Some case reports have described positive findings after chemotherapy and radiation therapy.[56–58] Those findings support the idea that sarcoidosis is an immune system disease and can flare up when the immune system is compromised. Yao and colleagues[57] reported that a patient showed abnormal FDG uptake in the neck and mediastinum after intensity-modulated radiation therapy. The pretreatment PET scan was normal in the chest, and biopsy showed granulomatous changes with necrosis.

The authors' own experience supports these reported findings.

FDG PET scan is valuable in evaluating pulmonary sarcoidosis and extrapulmonary involvement of the disease.[10,36] A case from Fox Chase Cancer Center shows the full extent of the disease detected by PET study (Fig. 4). FDG PET scan is also valuable in detecting unsuspected sites of involvement, leading to successful diagnosis and therapy. A recent report by Cheng and colleagues[59] showed the rapid progression of mediastinal adenopathy in sarcoidosis. This finding is likely a result of the high-contrast resolution of the PET scan, with semiquantitative analysis. Another management review by Braun and colleagues[60] concluded that 18F-FDG PET/CT allows clinicians to obtain a complete morphofunctional cartography of inflammatory active localizations and to follow treatment efficacy in patients with sarcoidosis, particularly in atypical, complex, and multisystemic forms.

PET/CT is also of value in monitoring treatment response and in deciding to whether continue the present treatment or switch to an alternate therapeutic regimen.[61–63] In an observation study of 12 patients treated with infliximab for sarcoid by FDG-PET scans, Keijsers and coworks[64] found that the FDG uptake represents disease activity and correlates with clinical course. Another article[65] reported the early documentation (6 weeks) of therapy response using PET scans. In the patient shown in Fig. 1 with colorectal cancer at Fox Chase Cancer Center, the follow-up PET/CT scan performed 3 months later because of elevated carcinoembryonic antigen (CEA) showed progression of cancer with new lesions in the liver. However, the sarcoidosis showed slight regression with lower metabolic intensity (Fig. 5).

Brudin and coworkers[66] introduced a new concept for assessing regional pulmonary glucose metabolism (MRglu) as an index of the degree of inflammation, and have related it to other tests, such as routine pulmonary function tests, chest radiography, and serum angiotensin converting enzyme (SACE) levels. MRglu was measured in a single midthoracic transaxial slice using PET in seven patients with histologically proven sarcoidosis before and after high-dose steroid therapy. The authors concluded that MRglu measured with FDG-PET may reflect disease activity in sarcoidosis in quantitative terms (per gram lung tissue) and may correspond to disease distribution. The efficacy of this approach should be verified and validated in a large population study before it is adopted for routine use.

Milman and colleagues[67] used FDG PET to investigate temporal changes in disease activity

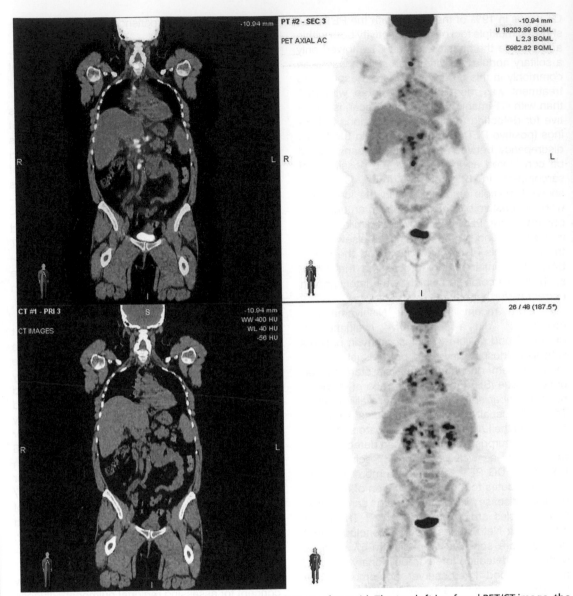

Fig. 4. PET/CT evaluation of a 48-year-old woman with history of sarcoid. The top left is a fused PET/CT image, the top right is a PET image, the bottom left is a CT image, and all images are in coronal display. The bottom right is a maximum-intensity projection image of the whole-body PET in posterior projection. In addition to the lesions in the mediastinum and right thorax laterally, active nodes are seen in the upper abdomen.

in a patient with pulmonary sarcoidosis before and during therapy with inhaled corticosteroids, followed by systemic administration of this drug. FDG PET was performed at baseline, 10 months, and 14 months after treatment. Before the second PET, the patient was treated with inhaled corticosteroid (beclomethasone) and before the third PET, the patient was treated with oral prednisolone. The first PET showed high FDG uptake in the hilar and mediastinal lymph nodes and in the pulmonary parenchyma and pleura. The second PET showed reduced uptake in the mediastinal

lymph nodes but seemed unchanged in the lungs and the pleura. However, the third PET showed no evidence of active disease. They concluded that based on FDG-PET, inhaled corticosteroids had no recognizable influence on inflammatory disease activity. In contrast, treatment with oral prednisolone reduced disease activity, as shown on PET. These data are concordant with clinical studies that show marginal effect from inhaled corticosteroids and a marked response from systemic administration of prednisolone. This study suggests that PET is a useful tool for testing

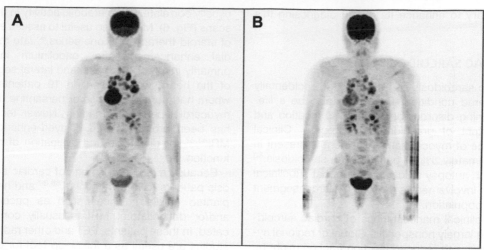

Fig. 5. The same patient in **Fig. 1**; a 57-year-old white woman with history of colorectal cancer and elevated car-cinoembryonic antigen referred for PET/CT follow-up. Both the previous scan (A) and the current scan (B) are maximum-intensity projection images in posterior projection. The SUV in the current scan is 5.1 in the left and 6.3 in the right, compared with the prior scan, in which is 7.3 in the left and 8.0 in the right.

the efficacy of various treatments and the optimal route for administering the drugs.

In addition to FDG, other PET tracers have been used to evaluate sarcoidosis and other granulomatous diseases.[68] Hain and coworkers[68] used C-11–labeled methionine to evaluate granulomatous disease. The short half-life of C-11 is a main hurdle for widespread use of this tracer. Halter and coworkers[69] studied thymidine analog 3'-deoxy-3'[(18)F]fluorothymidine (FLT) and compared the results with those of FDG PET scan. FLT is a tracer that specifically targets proliferative activity of malignant and noncancerous cells. This prospective study was performed during preoperative workup with subsequent pathologic correlations. The preliminary findings indicated that, compared with FDG, FLT uptake is specific for malignant lesions and reveals fewer false-positive findings in patients with sarcoidosis.

Yamada and colleagues[70] conducted a study in which C-11 methionine (MET) was used to evaluate mediastinal and hilar lymph nodes in 31 patients with sarcoidosis. The study was designed to examine and define the role of FDG PET and C-11-MET PET in the clinical assessment of pulmonary involvement of this disease. These scans were performed within a few days of each other. The differential uptake ratio of these tracers was calculated for the region of interest with the most intense activity. All patients had a minimum of 1-year follow-up, which included a clinical reassessment. In repeat imaging studies conducted on seven patients, lymph nodes remained visible. The investigators also calculated the FDG/MET uptake ratios and divided patients into FDG-dominant

(FDG/MET uptake ratio≥2) and MET-dominant groups (FDG/MET uptake ratio<2). They noted that the rate of improvement assessed through clinical findings and chest radiographs correlated considerably better with the FDG-dominant (78%) than the MET-dominant groups (33%). In the seven patients with repeated PET examinations, the FDG/MET uptake ratios seemed unchanged after 1 year. The authors concluded that the FDG/MET uptake ratio on PET studies may reflect the differential granulomatous state in this disorder.

Kaira and colleagues[71] evaluated the diagnostic usefulness of F18-alpha-methyltyrosine (FMT) PET in combination with FDG PET for patients with sarcoidosis. The mechanism for the novel tracer is an analog of amino acid transporter, and patients with sarcoidosis showed no increased FMT uptake. For patients with cancer as control, FMT scan showed increased activity. The conclusion is to use both scans to differentiate sarcoidosis from malignancy. This may be useful in certain populations of patients with both sarcoid and another concurrent malignancy.[72–79] Because of the complexity of the scans and high cost of imaging with dual tracers, these multiradiotracer studies have not gained widespread acceptance in clinical practice.

Overall, these data indicate that FDG as a single tracer is superior to the other existing agents for managing patients with sarcoidosis. Therefore, FDG PET as a single modality seems promising for the detection, full-extent evaluation, and follow-up of disease activity in sarcoidosis. However, well-designed prospective clinical trials are necessary to enhance its role in diagnosing this disease.

CARDIAC SARCOIDOSIS

Cardiac sarcoidosis can be a benign, incidentally discovered condition. But it can also be a life-threatening disorder because of its location and the extent of granulomatous process. Clinical evidence of myocardial involvement is present in approximately 5% of patients with sarcoidosis,[80] although autopsy studies indicate that subclinical cardiac involvement is present in a larger segment of this population.[81]

The clinical manifestations of cardiac sarcoidosis are largely nonspecific. Global or regional hypokinesis with reduced ejection fraction might be present. The findings in echocardiogram can be either systolic dysfunction with reduced contraction, diastolic dysfunction with dilated left ventricular chamber, or both. Echocardiogram is operator-dependent and not sensitive for detecting focal disease.[82] Myocardial involvement is common in patients with sarcoidosis who have cardiac symptoms and unusual in those without these symptoms. For definitive diagnosis, endomyocardial biopsy may be required, which is an established diagnostic procedure. However, sampling error may produce false-negative results because myocardial involvement may be nonuniform.

Chest radiography may reveal nonspecific findings, such as mild to moderate cardiomegaly, congestive heart failure, pericardial effusion, or a left ventricular aneurysm. The findings could be seen in combination with or without pulmonary sarcoidosis at various stages. In a case series by Milman and colleagues,[83] eight patients were treated for cardiac sarcoidosis with various signs and symptoms: two patients had heart block, five ventricular arrhythmias, and six had dilated cardiomyopathy with congestive heart failure. Diagnosis was very difficult: three patients were diagnosed with endomyocardial biopsy, three at heart transplantation (HTx), and two at autopsy.

Cardiac MRI is a new and noninvasive modality, with considerable improvement in the diagnosis and monitoring myocardial sarcoidosis over the years with increased experience. A variety of findings have been noted, including localized cardiac scar and high-intensity areas on T1- and/or T2-weighted images. Gadolinium-diethylene-triamine penta-acetic acid (DTPA) enhancement permits early detection of cardiac involvement through allowing direct visualization of the contrast accumulation, and provides better sensitivity and structural characterization of the lesions.[82] MRI findings usually correlate with metabolic activity in the PET scans (**Fig. 6**). MRI is also useful to assess efficacy of steroid therapy.[84] In one series,[85] late myocardial enhancement after gadolinium infusion, primarily involving the basal and lateral segments of the heart, was present in 19 patients, 8 of whom had normal exercise or persantine thallium myocardial perfusion imaging. Newer technique has been proposed with delayed-enhancement MRI[86,87] for diagnosis and evaluation of cardiac function.

Because a high percentage of cardiac sarcoidosis patients have arrhythmias,[88,89] and have implanted cardiac devices such as pacemakers and/or defibrillators, MRI is usually contraindicated. In these patients, PET and other radiotracer studies are useful as a follow-up tool for disease monitoring.[90–92] MRI-safe devices have become more prevalent in recent years, but clinicians and patients are hesitant to perform MRI scan because of the concerns. In these cases, functional imaging with radionuclides and PET tracers can be more suitable (**Fig. 7**).

The role of cardiac catheterization and coronary angiography is limited in diagnosing sarcoidosis, but thrombosis, aneurysm formation, and partial or complete narrowing of the epicardial coronary arteries from sarcoidosis can be visualized with these techniques.

Conventional cardiac nuclear medicine procedures, such as thallium 201– and Tc 99m–labeled myocardial perfusion scans, may be helpful in patients with suspected cardiac sarcoidosis to determine myocardial or coronary artery involvement. For patients who have known systemic sarcoidosis, perfusion defects will strongly suggest cardiac involvement if atherosclerotic coronary disease is excluded as the underlying cause of these abnormalities. Decreased perfusion in the ventricular wall usually corresponds to the areas of fibrogranulomatous tissue replacement.

A thallium perfusion study is useful for monitoring response to treatment in patients with myocardial sarcoidosis.[93] The tracer and imaging technique are well established, but the efficacy of this technique for this indication is not as common.

Okayama and coworkers[94] proposed using a combination of cardiac perfusion and gallium-67 imaging to diagnose and monitor cardiac sarcoidosis. The investigators believe that this combination may improve the ability to detect cardiac sarcoidosis. In this study, half of the patients with abnormal perfusion showed increased gallium-67 uptake. This report suggests that gallium-positive lesions may respond to corticosteroids, and that this treatment may therefore improve myocardial function.

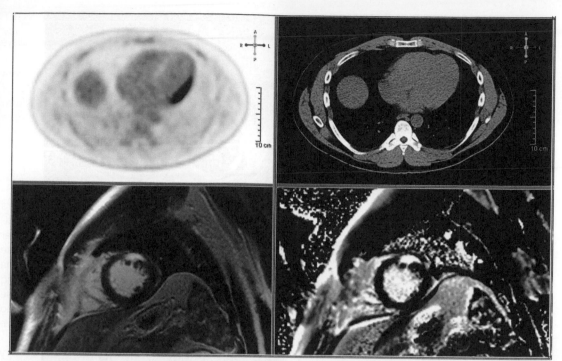

Fig. 6. PET/CT scan to evaluate myocardial involvement in a 37-year-old man with sarcoidosis. No prior PET scans were available for comparison. Images were acquired from just below the thoracic inlet to the upper abdomen 59 minutes postinjection of 14.4 mCi 18F-FDG. The blood glucose before injection was 112 mg/dL. The images showed intense focal activity in the anterolateral wall of the left ventricle with a maximum SUV of 7.8. An MRI examination of the chest was performed at 1.5 T, with attention directed toward evaluation of the heart using a variety of pulse sequences, including multiplanar black blood, cine bright blood True Fast Imaging With Steady-State Acquisition (TrueFISP), phase contrast, postcontrast perfusion, and delayed images. The MR images show delayed enhancement in the left ventricular myocardium, better seen in the anterolateral wall of the left ventricle where the enhancement is essentially full thickness.

The role of F18-FDG PET imaging in cardiac sarcoidosis is controversial. A case report describes the usefulness of PET study in the detection of cardiac sarcoidosis.[95] Mehta and colleagues[82] believe that PET is more sensitive for detection than current established criteria used for routine clinical assessment. Another group studied the pattern of FDG uptake in patients with known cardiac sarcoidosis[96] and concluded that focal uptake is a typical feature in this setting. This study also reported a crude comparison between FDG PET and other nuclear medicine studies, such as gallium-67 and Tc 99m sestamibi scan. The results showed that FDG PET can detect cardiac sarcoidosis when gallium-67 or Tc 99m MIBI scintigraphy appears negative. Another study confirmed these findings.[97]

Other studies showed that fasting FDG PET can detect early inflammation from cardiac sarcoidosis, before the development of advanced fibrosis.[98–101] The combination of the MRI and PET may improve the required information for optimal management of these patients.[102–106] Cardiac sarcoid can occur with pulmonary and mediastinal sarcoidosis (**Fig. 8**). When interpreting the PET study with lung sarcoidosis, one should be aware of the patchy and focal activity in the myocardium, which indicates heart involvement.[107]

Ohira and coworkers[108] performed myocardial imaging with FDG PET and MRI in sarcoidosis. They found that both modalities are sensitive for diagnosing cardiac involvement by sarcoid. PET correlated with elevated serum angiotensin-converting enzyme (ACE) levels, not the MRI. Those results suggest that PET may be better for active disease and would be more useful for following treatment response. Inflammatory activity assessment[109] is the latest indication for research. Another recent article by Basu and colleagues[110] also explored the relationship between PET and serum ACE level. PET scan has multiple technical issues, especially patient preparation with fasting,[111] longer fasting,[112] and

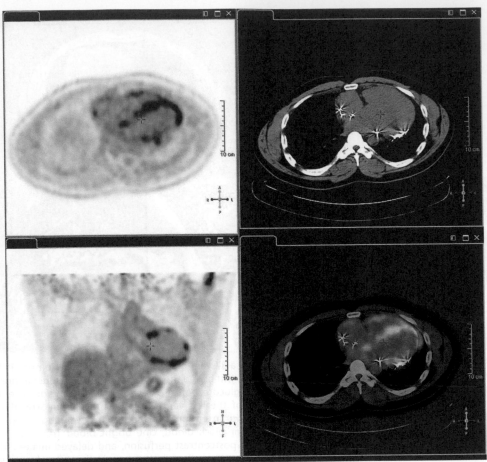

Fig. 7. FDG PET study to assess myocardial involvement in a 47-year-old man with clinical history of sarcoidosis and ventricular tachycardia after placement of an implantable cardioverter defibrillator. The study was performed after the patient was put on a low-carbohydrate, high-fat/protein diet. The blood glucose at the time of injection was 119 mg/dL. Images of the chest and upper abdomen were acquired 80 minutes postinjection of 15 mCi of 18F-FDG. Axial, sagittal (not shown), and coronal PET reconstructions with attenuation correction were interpreted. Persistent patchy heterogeneous uptake involving most of the left ventricular myocardium is seen on the prior scan, with interval improvement only in some regions of the inferior left ventricular wall. Residual patchy activity is also noted in the right ventricular wall. Mild persistent FDG activity is seen in the bilateral perihilar region.

gated acquisition,[113] which requires special attention and standardization.

Yamagishi and colleagues[114] used both N13-NH3 for perfusion and F18-FDG PET for metabolism in assessing disease activity. They showed equivalent sensitivity for both tests, but FDG PET seemed superior for monitoring treatment response and may be advantageous over conventional nuclear medicine studies, such as thallium-201 and gallium-67 scans in this setting. However, false-negative results have been noted with this technique.[102] A patient with known active cardiac sarcoid and structural changes shown by other tests failed to show abnormal activity in either gallium-67 or PET scan. Therefore, further research is needed to define the role of PET in cardiac sarcoidosis. Isiguzo and colleagues[115] proposed another method of perfusion and metabolism coupling with rubidium-FDG dual-tracer PET. Miwa and coworkers[116] compared of FDG PET with carbon-11–labeled choline PET for early detection of cardiac sarcoidosis. The result is encouraging, but the clinical utility of carbon-11–labeled compound is limited because of short half-life of the tracer (20 minutes). It might be useful in only academic settings that have an onsite cyclotron.

NEUROSARCOIDOSIS

Neurologic complications occur in approximately 5% of patients with sarcoidosis.[117] Neurosarcoidosis

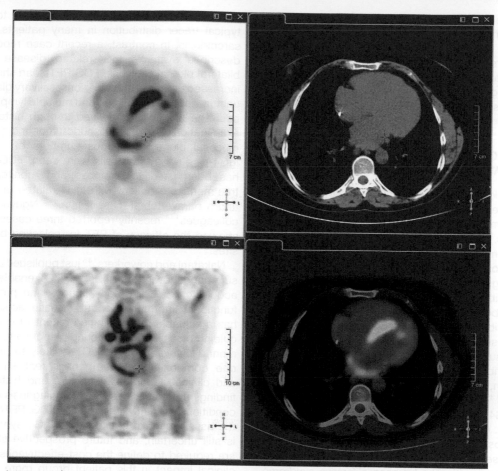

Fig. 8. Images ordered to evaluate for myocardial involvement of sarcoidosis in a 59-year-old woman with sarcoidosis. Blood glucose level before injection was 107 mg/dL. Images were acquired from the lower neck to the upper abdomen approximately 1 hour after the injection of 14.7 mCi 18F-FDG. Axial, coronal, and sagittal (not shown) PET reconstructions were interpreted with attenuation correction. In addition to mediastinal and bilateral hilar lymphadenopathy, increased radiotracer uptake is seen with a maximum SUV of 10.0 in the left ventricular myocardium, with most intensity at the anterior base. Again, a significant amount of septal involvement is seen with a maximum SUV of 11.1.

is a diagnostic dilemma in patients with known sarcoidosis who develop neurologic complaints, and in patients presenting de novo with a constellation of findings consistent with the disease. Approximately 50% of patients with eventual diagnosis of neurosarcoidosis present with neurologic difficulties at initial diagnosis of the disease. One-third of those with neurosarcoidosis will develop more than one neurologic manifestation of the disease.

The preferred imaging procedure for the diagnosis of central nervous system sarcoidosis is contrast-enhanced MRI. Meningeal or parenchymal enhancement suggests active inflammation with disruption of the blood–brain barrier with or without mass effects and hydrocephalus. Involvement of the optic nerve or other cranial nerves can be documented, and spinal cord and cauda equina inflammation is well seen on targeted anatomic images.

If the diagnosis remains in doubt, meningeal, brain, or spinal cord biopsy is occasionally indicated. Performing a biopsy to establish the diagnosis, rather than initiating an empiric therapy, should be considered if no evidence of systemic disease is present. Muscle and peripheral nerve biopsy can be easily performed if clinically warranted.

Reports related to the role of nuclear medicine procedure in neurosarcoidosis are scarce in the literature. One author[118] suggested that FDG PET might be helpful in overcoming some of the limitations of MRI. Other case reports of neurosarcoidosis[119–123] describe certain findings related to this disorder that reveal incidental findings with this technique.[124] One case series recently reported[125] has only six patients, and all have pathologic confirmation in addition to PET scan. The authors advocate the use of PET scan to evaluate any patients suspected of having neurosarcoidosis. In general, PET is helpful for detecting clinically silent sites and directing biopsy to the appropriate site for definitive diagnosis anywhere in the body.

SARCOID IN OTHER ORGANS AND IgG4 DISEASE

Sarcoidosis is a systemic disease and could involve any organs/systems. Musculoskeletal system involvement is seen in up to 10% of the cases.[126] Plain radiographs and MRI are the two main modalities that are commonly used for the diagnosis of musculoskeletal sarcoidosis, but the findings are nonspecific. Case reports have described FDG uptake in the muscle,[127,128] and bone sarcoidosis.[129] Other authors have described PET findings in cervical lymph node sracoidosis,[130] bone marrow,[131,132] spine,[133] skin, and subcutaneous lesions.[134,135] Several articles describe the sarcoidosis in the head and neck region, including eyes,[136,137] lacrimal glands,[138] ears,[139] and larynx.[140]

IgG4 disease or syndrome is newly identified entity. Other terms, such as *IgG4-related systemic sclerosing disease*, *IgG4-related autoimmune disease*, *IgG4-related systemic disease*, and *IgG4-positive multiorgan lymphoproliferative syndrome*, have been used to identify the disease. The clinical manifestations are variable: sclerosing pancreatitis, sclerosing cholangitis, prostatitis, tubulointerstitial nephritis, interstitial pneumonia, and enlargement of salivary glands. These clinical entities were considered unrelated. However, recent studies showed that these conditions share some common denominators, such as elevated serum IgG4 levels and tissue infiltration by IgG4-positive plasma cells, accompanied by tissue fibrosis and sclerosis.

The patient population is mainly middle-aged men and usually has more than two organs involved simultaneously, including the pancreas (the most commonly affected tissue), gall bladder, bile duct, salivary glands, retroperitoneum, kidneys, lung, prostate, lymph nodes, breast, thyroid, and pituitary glands. Diagnosis of this syndrome depends on clinicians' awareness, blood IgG4 levels, and tissue biopsy. Most current literatures are from Japan and Asia with specific ethnic groups.

The FDG distribution in patients with IgG4 disease has not been well defined. Liu and colleagues[141] described their findings of FDG PET/CT in a patient with IgG4 disease. This patient had intense FDG activity in both hilar regions and

in the mediastinum, which is very similar to the typical tracer distribution in many patients with sarcoidosis. In contrast, a recent case report[142] describes systemic IgG4-related disease with bilateral pleural effusions. FDG PET scan showed increased uptake in orbital lesions, salivary glands, gastric wall, biliary system, and multiple lymph nodes. The diagnosis is derived through histologic examination of an orbital pseudotumor and gastric mucosal biopsy; numerous numbers of mostly IgG4-positive plasma cells were seen. FDG PET has been used to diagnose and monitor the treatment of a patient with IgG4-related disease and a paravertebral mass lesion.[143] Nguyen and colleagues[144] recently reported three cases, and showed the efficacy of PET for selecting biopsy sites.

Nakatani and coworkers[145] just published a brief summary showing that FDG PET/CT enables the acquisition of whole-body images and provides functional information about disease activity; it has a valuable role in staging extent of disease, guiding biopsy, and monitoring response to treatment. However, FDG PET/CT is likely to be only one component of the management strategy, and clinical, laboratory, imaging, and histologic findings are crucial in the overall diagnosis of the condition. Currently, the role of FDG PET/CT in the assessment of patients with IgG4 syndrome is still uncertain, and future prospective studies are required to define the cost-effectiveness and clinical impact in this patient group more accurately. Nevertheless, recognizing the pattern of the FDG distribution in the IgG4 disease is likely helpful in differentiating IgG4 disease from diseases with similar FDG PET/CT findings, such as sarcoidosis[36,75] or lymphoma.[146,147]

SUMMARY

PET scans are useful in the management of patients with sarcoidosis. The state-of-the-art PET/CT scan is even more helpful for evaluating the full extent of the disease. Whole-body imaging with PET allows detection of clinically silent sites, or unsuspected lesions, and identification of the sites for biopsy. The CT portion of the study is helpful for localizing the lesions and reducing false results. FDG PET is particularly useful for monitoring response to treatment and shows early response in advance of anatomic changes. PET/CT is complimentary with MRI in the evaluation of cardiac sarcoidosis and neurosarcoidosis. It has potential use for IgG4 disease because the syndrome has multiorgan involvement. Prospective well-designed research studies with larger cohorts are still required to further determine the role of this powerful modality in the management of these common disorders.

REFERENCES

1. Hutchinson J. Case of livid papillary psoriasis. Illustrations of Clinical Surgery. London: J and A Churchill; 1877. p. 42.

2. Rybicki BA, Major M, Popovich J Jr, et al. Racial differences in sarcoidosis incidence: a 5-year study in a health maintenance organization. Am J Epidemiol 1997;145:234–41.

3. Revsbech P. Is sarcoidosis related to exposure to pets or the housing conditions? A case-referent study. Sarcoidosis 1992;9:101–3.

4. Sulavik SB, Spencer RP, Weed DA, et al. Recognition of distinctive patterns of gallium-67 distribution in sarcoidosis. J Nucl Med 1990;31:1909–14.

5. Tada A. [67Gallium whole body scintigraphy and single photon emission computed tomography (SPECT) in sarcoidosis]. Nihon Rinsho 2002;60: 1753–8 [in Japanese].

6. Shorr AF, Helman DL, Lettieri CJ, et al. Depreotide scanning in sarcoidosis: a pilot study. Chest 2004; 126:1337–43.

7. Lebtahi R, Crestani B, Belmatoug N, et al. Somatostatin receptor scintigraphy and gallium scintigraphy in patients with sarcoidosis. J Nucl Med 2001;42:21–6.

8. Alavi A, Buchpiguel CA, Loessner A. Is there a role for FDG PET imaging in the management of patients with sarcoidosis? J Nucl Med 1994;35: 1650–2.

9. Yu JQ, Zhuang H, Xiu Y, et al. Demonstration of increased FDG activity in Rosai-Dorfman disease on positron emission tomography. Clin Nucl Med 2004;29:209–10.

10. El-Haddad G, Zhuang H, Gupta N, et al. Evolving role of positron emission tomography in the management of patients with inflammatory and other benign disorders. Semin Nucl Med 2004;34:313–29.

11. Yu JQ, Kung JW, Potenta S, et al. Chronic cholecystitis detected by FDG-PET. Clin Nucl Med 2004;29:496–7.

12. Zhuang H, Yu JQ, Alavi A. Applications of fluorodeoxyglucose-PET imaging in the detection of infection and inflammation and other benign disorders. Radiol Clin North Am 2005;43:121–34.

13. Yu JQ, Kumar R, Xiu Y, et al. Diffuse FDG uptake in the lungs in aspiration pneumonia on positron emission tomographic imaging. Clin Nucl Med 2004;29:567–8.

14. Alavi A, Gupta N, Alberini JL, et al. Positron emission tomography imaging in nonmalignant thoracic disorders. Semin Nucl Med 2002;32:293–321.

15. Kung J, Zhuang H, Yu JQ, et al. Intense fluorodeoxyglucose activity in pulmonary amyloid lesions on positron emission tomography. Clin Nucl Med 2003;28:975–6.

16. Zhuang H, Alavi A. 18-fluorodeoxyglucose positron emission tomographic imaging in the detection and monitoring of infection and inflammation. Semin Nucl Med 2002;32:47–59.

17. Nguyen BD. F-18 FDG PET imaging of disseminated sarcoidosis. Clin Nucl Med 2007;32:53–4.

18. Tannen BL, Ghesani NV, Frohman L, et al. Use of whole-body FDG PET-CT to aid in the diagnosis of occult sarcoidosis. Ocul Immunol Inflamm 2008;16:25–7.

19. Seve P, Billotey C, Janier M, et al. Fluorodeoxyglucose positron emission tomography for the diagnosis of sarcoidosis in patients with unexplained chronic uveitis. Ocul Immunol Inflamm 2009;17: 179–84.

20. Ambrosini V, Fasano L, Zompatori M, et al. (18)F-FDG PET/CT detects systemic involvement in sarcoidosis. Eur J Nucl Med Mol Imaging 2011; 14:311–2.

21. Teirstein AS, Machac J, Almeida O, et al. Results of 188 whole-body fluorodeoxyglucose positron emission tomography scans in 137 patients with sarcoidosis. Chest 2007;132:1949–53.

22. Lewis PJ, Salama A. Uptake of fluorine-18-fluorodeoxyglucose in sarcoidosis. J Nucl Med 1994;35:1647–9.

23. Larson SM. Cancer or inflammation? a holy grail for nuclear medicine. J Nucl Med 1994;35:1653–5.

24. Muggia FM, Conti PS. Seminoma and sarcoidosis: a cause for false positive mediastinal uptake in PET? Ann Oncol 1998;9:924.

25. Yasuda S, Shohtsu A, Ide M, et al. High fluorine-18 labeled deoxyglucose uptake in sarcoidosis. Clin Nucl Med 1996;21:983–4.

26. Ataergin S, Arslan N, Ozet A, et al. Abnormal 18F-FDG uptake detected with positron emission tomography in a patient with breast cancer: a case of sarcoidosis and review of the literature. Case Report Med 2009;2009:785047.

27. Kiatboonsri C, Resnick SC, Chan KM, et al. The detection of recurrent sarcoidosis by FDG-PET in a lung transplant recipient. West J Med 1998;168: 130–2.

28. Gotway MB, Storto ML, Golden JA, et al. Incidental detection of thoracic sarcoidosis on whole-body 18fluorine-2- fluoro-2-deoxy-D-glucose positron emission tomography. J Thorac Imaging 2000;15: 201–4.

29. Takanami K, Kaneta T, Yamada T, et al. FDG PET for esophageal cancer complicated by sarcoidosis mimicking mediastinal and hilar lymph node metastases: two case reports. Clin Nucl Med 2008;33:258–61.

30. Kunstmann L, Bstandig B, Brucker-Davis F, et al. Malignant struma ovarii: false positive PET image

for suspected metastasis due to sarcoidosis. Ann Endocrinol (Paris) 2007;68:51–4 [in French].

31. Subbiah V, Ly UK, Khiyami A, et al. Tissue is the issue-sarcoidosis following ABVD chemotherapy for Hodgkin's lymphoma: a case report. J Med Case Reports 2007;1:148.

32. Itoh T, Kobayashi D, Rensha K, et al. A case of sarcoidosis presenting as a solitary pulmonary nodule. Nihon Kokyuki Gakkai Zasshi 2008;46: 992–6 [in Japanese].

33. Kruger S, Buck AK, Mottaghy FM, et al. Use of integrated FDG-PET/CT in sarcoidosis. Clin Imaging 2008;32:269–73.

34. Chida M, Inoue T, Honma K, et al. Sarcoid-like reaction mimics progression of disease after induction chemotherapy for lung cancer. Ann Thorac Surg 2010;90:2031–3.

35. Kumar A, Dutta R, Kannan U, et al. Evaluation of mediastinal lymph nodes using F-FDG PET-CT scan and its histopathologic correlation. Ann Thorac Med 2011;6:11–6.

36. Xiu Y, Yu JQ, Cheng E, et al. Sarcoidosis demonstrated by FDG PET imaging with negative findings on gallium scintigraphy. Clin Nucl Med 2005;30: 193–5.

37. Nishiyama Y, Yamamoto Y, Fukunaga K, et al. Comparative evaluation of 18F-FDG PET and 67Ga scintigraphy in patients with sarcoidosis. J Nucl Med 2006;47:1571–6.

38. Carbone R, Douroukas A, Arena V, et al. Does 18F-fluorodeoxyglucose PET/CT have a role in the management of pulmonary and extra pulmonary sarcoidosis? Monaldi Arch Chest Dis 2008;69: 81–2.

39. Prager E, Wehrschuetz M, Bisail B, et al. Comparison of 18F-FDG and 67Ga-citrate in sarcoidosis imaging. Nuklearmedizin 2008;47:18–23.

40. Keijsers RG, Grutters JC, Thomeer M, et al. Imaging the inflammatory activity of sarcoidosis: sensitivity and inter observer agreement of (67) Ga imaging and (18)F-FDG PET. Q J Nucl Med Mol Imaging 2011;55:66–71.

41. Arfi J, Kerrou K, Traore S, et al. F-18 FDG PET/CT findings in pulmonary necrotizing sarcoid granulomatosis. Clin Nucl Med 2010;35:697–700.

42. Keijsers RG, Grutters JC, van Velzen-Blad H, et al. (18)F-FDG PET patterns and BAL cell profiles in pulmonary sarcoidosis. Eur J Nucl Med Mol Imaging 2010;37:1181–8.

43. van der Veldt AA, Comans EF, Thunnissen FB, et al. Re: sarcoid-like reaction to malignancy on whole-body integrated 18F-FDG PET/CT: prevalence and disease pattern. Clin Radiol 2010;65:94–6 [author reply: 96–7].

44. Kubota K, Itoh M, Ozaki K, et al. Advantage of delayed whole-body FDG-PET imaging for tumour detection. Eur J Nucl Med 2001;28:696–703.

45. Cremerius U, Wildberger JE, Borchers H, et al. Does positron emission tomography using 18-fluoro-2-deoxyglucose improve clinical staging of testicular cancer?–results of a study in 50 patients. Urology 1999;54:900–4.

46. de Hemricourt E, De Boeck K, Hilte F, et al. Sarcoidosis and sarcoid-like reaction following Hodgkin's disease. Report of two cases. Mol Imaging Biol 2003;5:15–9.

47. Higashi K, Ueda Y, Sakuma T, et al. Comparison of [(18)F]FDG PET and (201)Tl SPECT in evaluation of pulmonary nodules. J Nucl Med 2001;42: 1489–96.

48. Kalff V, Hicks RJ, Ware RE, et al. The clinical impact of (18)F-FDG PET in patients with suspected or confirmed recurrence of colorectal cancer: a prospective study. J Nucl Med 2002;43:492–9.

49. Karapetis CS, Strickland AH, Yip D, et al. PET and PLAP in suspected testicular cancer relapse: beware sarcoidosis. Ann Oncol 2001;12:1485–8.

50. Kubota K, Yamada S, Kondo T, et al. PET imaging of primary mediastinal tumours. Br J Cancer 1996; 73:882–6.

51. Nguyen AT, Akhurst T, Larson SM, et al. PET Scanning with (18)F 2-Fluoro-2-Deoxy-D-Glucose (FDG) in patients with melanoma. Benefits and limitations. Clin Positron Imaging 1999;2:93–8.

52. Pitman AG, Hicks RJ, Binns DS, et al. Performance of sodium iodide based (18)F-fluorodeoxyglucose positron emission tomography in the characterization of indeterminate pulmonary nodules or masses. Br J Radiol 2002;75:114–21.

53. Pitman AG, Hicks RJ, Kalff V, et al. Positron emission tomography in pulmonary masses where tissue diagnosis is unhelpful or not possible. Med J Aust 2001;175:303–7.

54. van der Hoeven JJ, Krak NC, Hoekstra OS, et al. 18F-2-fluoro-2-deoxy-d-glucose positron emission tomography in staging of locally advanced breast cancer. J Clin Oncol 2004;22:1253–9.

55. Umezu H, Chida M, Inoue T, et al. Sarcoidosis development during induction chemotherapy for lung cancer mimicked progressive disease. Gen Thorac Cardiovasc Surg 2010;58:434–7.

56. Maeda J, Ohta M, Hirabayashi H, et al. False positive accumulation in 18F fluorodeoxyglucose positron emission tomography scan due to sarcoid reaction following induction chemotherapy for lung cancer. Jpn J Thorac Cardiovasc Surg 2005; 53:196–8.

57. Yao M, Funk GF, Goldstein DP, et al. Benign lesions in cancer patients: case 1. Sarcoidosis after chemoradiation for head and neck cancer. J Clin Oncol 2005;23:640–1.

58. Cherk MH, Pham A, Haydon A. 18F-fluorodeoxyglucose positron emission tomography-positive sarcoidosis after chemoradiotherapy for Hodgkin's

disease: a case report. J Med Case Reports 2011; 5:247.

59. Cheng CY, Huang WS, Shen DH, et al. FDG PET/CT demonstrated rapid progression of mediastinal lymphadenopathy in sarcoidosis. Clin Nucl Med 2007;32:117–21.

60. Braun JJ, Kessler R, Constantinesco A, et al. 18F-FDG PET/CT in sarcoidosis management: review and report of 20 cases. Eur J Nucl Med Mol Imaging 2008;35:1537–43.

61. Mortensen J, Loft A, Baslund B. 18F-fluoro-deoxy-glucose PET for monitoring treatment in sarcoidosis. Clin Respir J 2007;1:124–6.

62. Kaneko M, Tomioka H, Kaneda T, et al. [Value of 18F-fluorodeoxyglucose-PET in the diagonosis and monitoring of pulmonary sarcoidosis: a case report]. Nihon Kokyuki Gakkai Zasshi 2008;46: 505–9 [in Japanese].

63. Kaira K. [Usefulness of FDG-PET for monitoring the effects of therapy in sarcoidosis patients]. Nihon Kokyuki Gakkai Zasshi 2009;47:1166 [in Japanese] [author reply: 1167].

64. Keijsers RG, Verzijlbergen JF, van Diepen DM, et al. 18F-FDG PET in sarcoidosis: an observational study in 12 patients treated with infliximab. Sarcoidosis Vasc Diffuse Lung Dis 2008;25:143–9.

65. Basu S, Asopa RV, Baghel NS. Early documentation of therapeutic response at 6 weeks following corticosteroid therapy in extensive sarcoidosis: promise of FDG-PET. Clin Nucl Med 2009;34: 689–90.

66. Brudin LH, Valind SO, Rhodes CG, et al. Fluorine-18 deoxyglucose uptake in sarcoidosis measured with positron emission tomography. Eur J Nucl Med 1994;21:297–305.

67. Milman N, Mortensen J, Sloth C. Fluorodeoxyglucose PET scan in pulmonary sarcoidosis during treatment with inhaled and oral corticosteroids. Respiration 2003;70:408–13.

68. Hain SF, Beggs AD. C-11 methionine uptake in granulomatous disease. Clin Nucl Med 2004;29:585–6.

69. Halter G, Buck AK, Schirrmeister H, et al. [18F] 3-deoxy-3'-fluorothymidine positron emission tomography: alternative or diagnostic adjunct to 2-[18f]-fluoro-2-deoxy-D-glucose positron emission tomography in the workup of suspicious central focal lesions? J Thorac Cardiovasc Surg 2004; 127:1093–9.

70. Yamada Y, Uchida Y, Tatsumi K, et al. Fluorine-18-fluorodeoxyglucose and carbon-11-methionine evaluation of lymphadenopathy in sarcoidosis. J Nucl Med 1998;39:1160–6.

71. Kaira K, Oriuchi N, Otani Y, et al. Diagnostic usefulness of fluorine-18-alpha-methyltyrosine positron emission tomography in combination with 18F-fluorodeoxyglucose in sarcoidosis patients. Chest 2007;131:1019–27.

72. Chowdhury FU, Sheerin F, Bradley KM, et al. Sarcoid-like reaction to malignancy on whole-body integrated (18)F-FDG PET/CT: prevalence and disease pattern. Clin Radiol 2009;64:675–81.

73. Froio E, D'Adda T, Fellegara G, et al. Uterine carcinosarcoma metastatic to the lung as large-cell neuroendocrine carcinoma with synchronous sarcoid granulomatosis. Lung Cancer 2009;64: 371–7.

74. Gallagher DJ, Libby DM, Kemeny N. Elevated carcinoembryonic antigen and sarcoidosis masquerading as metastatic colon cancer. Clin Colorectal Cancer 2009;8:172–4.

75. Hunt BM, Vallieres E, Buduhan G, et al. Sarcoidosis as a benign cause of lymphadenopathy in cancer patients. Am J Surg 2009;197:629–32 [discussion: 632].

76. Costabel U, Bonella F, Ohshimo S, et al. Diagnostic modalities in sarcoidosis: BAL, EBUS, and PET. Semin Respir Crit Care Med 2010;31:404–8.

77. Schauer M, Theisen J. The diagnostic challenge of mediastinal sarcoidosis accompanying esophageal cancer. World J Surg Oncol 2010;8:15.

78. Urushiyama H, Yamauchi Y, Suzuki S, et al. [Case of sarcoidosis with squamous cell carcinoma which originated from solitary bronchial papilloma]. Nihon Kokyuki Gakkai Zasshi 2010;48:815–20 [in Japanese].

79. Cioffi U, Raveglia F, De Simone M, et al. Multiple right-sided pulmonary nodules: metastatic cancer or resectable early stage tumor? J Cardiothorac Surg 2011;6:105.

80. Hunninghake GW, Costabel U, Ando M, et al. ATS/ERS/WASOG statement on sarcoidosis. American Thoracic Society/European Respiratory Society/World Association of Sarcoidosis and other Granulomatous Disorders. Sarcoidosis Vasc Diffuse Lung Dis 1999;16:149–73.

81. Matsui Y, Iwai K, Tachibana T, et al. Clinicopathological study of fatal myocardial sarcoidosis. Ann N Y Acad Sci 1976;278:455–69.

82. Mehta D, Lubitz SA, Frankel Z, et al. Cardiac involvement in patients with sarcoidosis: diagnostic and prognostic value of outpatient testing. Chest 2008;133:1426–35.

83. Milman N, Andersen CB, Mortensen SA. [Cardiac sarcoidosis–a difficult diagnosis. A report of 8 consecutive patients with arrhythmias and cardiomyopathy]. Ugeskr Laeger 2006;168:3822–4 [in Danish].

84. Smedema JP, van Kroonenburgh MJ, Snoep G, et al. Diagnostic Value of PET in Cardiac Sarcoidosis. J Nucl Med 2004;45:1975.

85. Smedema JP, van Erven L, Schreur JH, et al. [Cardiac sarcoidosis: improved prognosis through new diagnostic tests and treatment]. Ned Tijdschr Geneeskd 2005;149:1168–73 [in Dutch].

86. Matoh F, Satoh H, Shiraki K, et al. The usefulness of delayed enhancement magnetic resonance imaging for diagnosis and evaluation of cardiac function in patients with cardiac sarcoidosis. J Cardiol 2008; 51:179–88.

87. Morrissey RP, Philip KJ, Schwarz ER. Reconciling Q waves and late gadolinium enhancement with no angiographic evidence of coronary disease: cardiac sarcoidosis presenting as decompensated heart failure. Cardiovasc J Afr 2010;21:158–63.

88. Miyazaki S, Funabashi N, Nagai T, et al. Cardiac sarcoidosis complicated with atrioventricular block and wall thinning, edema and fibrosis in left ventricle: confirmed recovery to normal sinus rhythm and visualization of edema improvement by administration of predonisolone. Int J Cardiol 2011;150:e4–10.

89. Thachil A, Christopher J, Sastry BK, et al. Monomorphic ventricular tachycardia and mediastinal adenopathy due to granulomatous infiltration in patients with preserved ventricular function. J Am Coll Cardiol 2011;58:48–55.

90. Gyorik S, Ceriani L, Menafoglio A, et al. 18F-FDG PET scan as follow-up tool for sarcoidosis with symptomatic cardiac conduction disturbances requiring a pacemaker. Thorax 2007;62:560.

91. Smedema JP, White L, Klopper AJ. FDG-PET and MIBI-Tc SPECT as follow-up tools in a patient with cardiac sarcoidosis requiring a pacemaker. Cardiovasc J Afr 2008;19:309–10.

92. Kruger S, Pauls S, Mottaghy FM, et al. [Cardiac sarcoidosis with 3rd degree AV block by means of integrated PET-CT]. Pneumologie 2007;61: 363–4 [in German].

93. Mana J. Nuclear imaging. 67Gallium, 201thallium, 18F-labeled fluoro-2-deoxy-D-glucose positron emission tomography. Clin Chest Med 1997;18:799–811.

94. Okayama K, Kurata C, Tawarahara K, et al. Diagnostic and prognostic value of myocardial scintigraphy with thallium-201 and gallium-67 in cardiac sarcoidosis. Chest 1995;107:330–4.

95. Goto K, Okamoto E, Morita M, et al. [Cardiac sarcoidosis detected by FDG-PET]. Nihon Naika Gakkai Zasshi 2005;94:1396–8 [in Japanese].

96. Ishimaru S, Tsujino I, Takei T, et al. Focal uptake on 18F-fluoro-2-deoxyglucose positron emission tomography images indicates cardiac involvement of sarcoidosis. Eur Heart J 2005;26:1538–43.

97. Nomura S, Funabashi N, Tsubura M, et al. Cardiac sarcoidosis evaluated by multimodality imaging. Int J Cardiol 2011;150:e81–4.

98. Okumura W, Iwasaki T, Toyama T, et al. Usefulness of fasting 18F FDG PET in identification of cardiac sarcoidosis. J Nucl Med 2004;45:1989–98.

99. Okumura W, Iwasaki T, Ueda T, et al. [Usefulness of 18F-FDG PET for diagnosis of cardiac sarcoidosis]. Kaku Igaku 1999;36:341–8 [in Japanese].

100. Ohira H, Tsujino I, Sato T, et al. Early detection of cardiac sarcoid lesions with (18)F-fluoro-2-deoxy-glucose positron emission tomography. Intern Med 2011;50:1207–9.

101. Ohira H, Tsujino I, Yoshinaga K. (1)F-Fluoro-2-deoxyglucose positron emission tomography in cardiac sarcoidosis. Eur J Nucl Med Mol Imaging 2011;38:1773–83.

102. Kaku B, Kanaya H, Horita Y, et al. Failure of follow-up gallium single-photon emission computed tomography and fluorine-18-fluorodeoxyglucose positron emission tomography to predict the deterioration of a patient with cardiac sarcoidosis. Circ J 2004;68:802–5.

103. Sharma S. Cardiac imaging in myocardial sarcoidosis and other cardiomyopathies. Curr Opin Pulm Med 2009;15:507–12.

104. Soejima K, Yada H. The work-up and management of patients with apparent or subclinical cardiac sarcoidosis: with emphasis on the associated heart rhythm abnormalities. J Cardiovasc Electrophysiol 2009;20:578–83.

105. Balan A, Hoey ET, Sheerin F, et al. Multi-technique imaging of sarcoidosis. Clin Radiol 2010;65: 750–60.

106. Imperiale A, Riehm S, Veillon F, et al. FDG PET coregistered to MRI for diagnosis and monitoring of therapeutic response in aggressive phenotype of sarcoidosis. Eur J Nucl Med Mol Imaging 2011; 38:983–4.

107. Tahara N, Tahara A, Nitta Y, et al. Heterogeneous myocardial FDG uptake and the disease activity in cardiac sarcoidosis. JACC Cardiovasc Imaging 2010;3:1219–28.

108. Ohira H, Tsujino I, Ishimaru S, et al. Myocardial imaging with 18F-fluoro-2-deoxyglucose positron emission tomography and magnetic resonance imaging in sarcoidosis. Eur J Nucl Med Mol Imaging 2008;35:933–41.

109. Mostard RL, Voo S, van Kroonenburgh MJ, et al. Inflammatory activity assessment by F18 FDG-PET/CT in persistent symptomatic sarcoidosis. Respir Med 2011;105(12):1917–24.

110. Basu S, Yadav M, Joshi JM, et al. Active pretreatment pure pulmonary parenchymal sarcoidosis with raised serum angiotensin converting enzyme level: characteristics on PET with glucose metabolism and cell proliferation tracers and HRCT. Eur J Nucl Med Mol Imaging 2011;38: 1584–5.

111. Brancato SC, Arrighi JA. Fasting FDG PET compared to MPI SPECT in cardiac sarcoidosis. J Nucl Cardiol 2011;18:371–4.

112. Langah R, Spicer K, Gehregziabher M, et al. Effectiveness of prolonged fasting 18f-FDG PET-CT in the detection of cardiac sarcoidosis. J Nucl Cardiol 2009;16:801–10.

113. Kokki T, Sipila HT, Teras M, et al. Dual gated PET/CT imaging of small targets of the heart: method description and testing with a dynamic heart phantom. J Nucl Cardiol 2010;17:71–84.

114. Yamagishi H, Shirai N, Takagi M, et al. Identification of cardiac sarcoidosis with (13)N-NH(3)/(18)F-FDG PET. J Nucl Med 2003;44:1030–6.

115. Isiguzo M, Brunken R, Tchou P, et al. Metabolism-perfusion imaging to predict disease activity in cardiac sarcoidosis. Sarcoidosis Vasc Diffuse Lung Dis 2011;28:50–5.

116. Miwa S, Inui N, Suda T, et al. Early detection of cardiac sarcoidosis: comparison of 18F-FDG PET with 11C-choline PET. Sarcoidosis Vasc Diffuse Lung Dis 2007;24:156–8.

117. Stern BJ. Neurological complications of sarcoidosis. Curr Opin Neurol 2004;17:311–6.

118. Braido F, Zolezzi A, Stea F, et al. Bilateral Gasser's ganglion sarcoidosis: diagnosis, treatment and unsolved questions. Sarcoidosis Vasc Diffuse Lung Dis 2005;22:75–7.

119. Dubey N, Miletich RS, Wasay M, et al. Role of fluorodeoxyglucose positron emission tomography in the diagnosis of neurosarcoidosis. J Neurol Sci 2002;205:77–81.

120. Ng D, Jacobs M, Mantil J. Combined C-11 methionine and F-18 FDG PET imaging in a case of neurosarcoidosis. Clin Nucl Med 2006;31:373–5.

121. Bolat S, Berding G, Dengler R, et al. Fluorodeoxyglucose positron emission tomography (FDG-PET) is useful in the diagnosis of neurosarcoidosis. J Neurol Sci 2009;287:257–9.

122. Yanagitani N, Kotake M, Ishizuka T, et al. A case of neurosarcoidosis discovered in a patient complaining of chest pain. Nihon Kokyuki Gakkai Zasshi 2009;47:1087–92 [in Japanese].

123. Kim SK, Im HJ, Kim W, et al. F-18 fluorodeoxyglucose and F-18 fluorothymidine positron emission tomography/computed tomography imaging in a case of neurosarcoidosis. Clin Nucl Med 2010;35:67–70.

124. Aide N, Benayoun M, Kerrou K, et al. Impact of [18F]-fluorodeoxyglucose ([18F]-FDG) imaging in sarcoidosis: unsuspected neurosarcoidosis discovered by [18F]-FDG PET and early metabolic response to corticosteroid therapy. Br J Radiol 2007;80:e67–71.

125. Magyari M, Frederiksen J. [Neurosarcoidosis—different manifestations]. Ugeskr Laeger 2010;172:3344–5 [in Danish].

126. Abril A, Cohen MD. Rheumatologic manifestations of sarcoidosis. Curr Opin Rheumatol 2004;16:51–5.

127. Dufour JF, Billotey C, Streichenberger N, et al. [Sarcoidosis demonstrated by fluorodeoxyglucose positron emission tomography in a case of granulomatous myopathy]. Rev Med Interne 2007;28:568–70 [in French].

128. Kolilekas L, Triantafillidou C, Manali E, et al. The many faces of sarcoidosis: asymptomatic muscle mass mimicking giant-cell tumor. Rheumatol Int 2009;29:1389–90.

129. Clarencon F, Silbermann-Hoffman O, Lebreton C, et al. Diffuse spine involvement in sarcoidosis with sternal lytic lesions: two case reports. Spine (Phila Pa 1976) 2007;32:E594–7.

130. Li YJ, Zhang Y, Gao S, et al. Cervical and axillary lymph node sarcoidosis misdiagnosed as lymphoma on F-18 FDG PET-CT. Clin Nucl Med 2007;32:262–4.

131. Baldini S, Pupi A, Di Lollo S, et al. PET positivity with bone marrow biopsy revealing sarcoidosis in a patient in whom bone marrow metastases had been suspected. Br J Haematol 2008;143:306.

132. de Prost N, Kerrou K, Sibony M, et al. Fluorine-18 fluorodeoxyglucose with positron emission tomography revealed bone marrow involvement in sarcoidosis patients with anaemia. Respiration 2010;79:25–31.

133. Ota K, Tsunemi T, Saito K, et al. 18F-FDG PET successfully detects spinal cord sarcoidosis. J Neurol 2009;256:1943–6.

134. Suarez-Garcia C, Perez-Gil A, Pereira-Gallardo S, et al. Interferon-induced cutaneous sarcoidosis in melanoma. Melanoma Res 2009;19:391–4.

135. Li Y, Berenji GR. Cutaneous sarcoidosis evaluated by FDG PET. Clin Nucl Med 2011;36:584–6.

136. Rahmi A, Deshayes E, Maucort-Boulch D, et al. Intraocular sarcoidosis: association of clinical characteristics of uveitis with findings from 18F-labelled fluorodeoxyglucose positron emission tomography. Br J Ophthalmol 2012;96(1):99–103.

137. Varron L, Abad S, Kodjikian L, et al. [Sarcoid uveitis: diagnostic and therapeutic update]. Rev Med Interne 2011;32:86–92 [in French].

138. Shulman JP, Latkany P, Chin KJ, et al. Whole-body 18FDG PET-CT imaging of systemic sarcoidosis: ophthalmic oncology and uveitis. Ocul Immunol Inflamm 2009;17:95–100.

139. Guedj E, Chiche L, Basely M, et al. 18FDG-PET/CT imaging of external ear sarcoidosis. Otol Neurotol 2010;31:699–700.

140. Kaira K, Ishizuka T, Yanagitani N, et al. Laryngeal sarcoidosis detected by FDG positron emission tomography. Clin Nucl Med 2008;33:878–9.

141. Liu Y, Chen L, Li F. Predominant IgG4 disease and concurrent early-stage rectal cancer. Clin Nucl Med 2011;36:1135–6.

142. A case of systemic IgG4-related disease with bilateral pleural effusions. Nihon Kokyuki Gakkai Zasshi 2011;49:214–20 [in Japanese].

143. Nakamura H, Hisatomi K, Koga T, et al. Successful treatment of a patient with IgG4-related disease with a paravertebral mass lesion. Mod Rheumatol 2011;21:524–7.

144. Nguyen VX, De Petris G, Nguyen BD. Usefulness of PET/CT imaging in systemic IgG4-related sclerosing disease. A report of three cases. JOP 2011;12:297–305.

145. Nakatani K, Nakamoto Y, Togashi K. Utility of FDG PET/CT in IgG4-related systemic disease. Clin Radiol 2011.

146. Elstrom R, Guan L, Baker G, et al. Utility of FDG-PET scanning in lymphoma by WHO classification. Blood 2003;101:3875–6.

147. Hernandez-Pampaloni M, Takalkar A, Yu JQ, et al. F-18 FDG-PET imaging and correlation with CT in staging and follow-up of pediatric lymphomas. Pediatr Radiol 2006;36:524–31.

Utilization of FDG PET/CT in the Management of Inflammation and Infection in Patients with Malignancies

Bing Xu, MD, PhD[a],*, Yuejian Liu, MD[a],
Ion Codreanu, MD, PhD[b]

KEYWORDS

- FDG-PET/CT • Inflammation • Infection • Malignancy

PET/COMPUTED TOMOGRAPHY AS AN EMERGING MODALITY FOR EVALUATION OF ASSOCIATED INFECTIONS IN PATIENTS WITH MALIGNANCY

Cancer has become one of the leading causes of death worldwide. Infections are common complications of malignancy, further contributing to the high mortality rate in these patients.[1] Many predisposing factors make patients with malignancies vulnerable to infection. The most common causes include disruption of the integrity of epidermal tissue or mucosal membranes by the tumor, obstruction of natural orifices, neutropenia caused by hematologic malignancies, bone marrow suppression after chemotherapy or immunosuppressive therapies, long-term administration of antibiotics or corticosteroids, invasive procedures, and prolonged hospitalization.[2,3] These alterations in the body's defense systems can predispose to a range of opportunistic infections, which may be life threatening. A weakened immune response frequently leads to atypical or faint clinical manifestations, further delaying the diagnosis of infection and increasing mortality. Among the most common entities, sepsis originating from respiratory tract infections accounts for almost half of the fatal outcomes.[4,5] Proper diagnosis is of utmost importance for early intervention in such situations. Conventional imaging, however, frequently fails to find a source of infection in patients with pyrexia or to differentiate malignant from infectious causes.[5,6] During recent decades, PET with 2-deoxy-2-[18F]fluoro-D-glucose (FDG) has emerged as a valuable imaging tool for diagnosis, staging, restaging, assessing the prognosis, and evaluating the response to therapy in a variety of tumors and hematologic malignancies.[7–11] It has been reported that PET imaging reveals unsuspected distal metastasis in about 10% to 15% of patients and leads to a change of therapy in 25% to 50% of patients.

The addition of the computed tomography (CT) component to PET yields several distinct advantages, for example, in the differential diagnosis of malignant and benign FDG uptake. Thus, lymph nodes meeting normal CT criteria (measuring <1 cm in short axis) may prove to be metabolically active on

[a] Department of Hematology, Nanfang Hospital, Southern Medical University, 1838 Guangzhou Avenue North, Guangzhou 510515, Guangdong Province, China
[b] Division of Nuclear Medicine, Department of Radiology, The Children's Hospital of Philadelphia, University of Pennsylvania School of Medicine, 34th Street and Civic Center Boulevard, Philadelphia, PA 19014, USA
* Corresponding author.
E-mail address: xubingzhangjian@126.com

PET Clin 7 (2012) 211–218
doi:10.1016/j.cpet.2012.01.008
1556-8598/12/$ – see front matter © 2012 Elsevier Inc. All rights reserved.

PET imaging. Conversely, enlarged lymph nodes or soft tissue masses may have little or no FDG uptake. Studies have shown that a PET/CT scan entails more accurate results compared with CT or PET alone or with side-by-side visual correlation of PET and CT scans.

Posttherapy PET/CT can provide valuable information for assessing treatment efficacy in many local and systemic infections such as sarcoidosis, vasculitis, tuberculosis, and aspergillosis. PET/CT has been used in such situations to adjust the drug dosage or to change the therapeutic strategy.[12] For this purpose, it is important to have a pretherapy scan and to standardize the scan protocols (prescan preparation, hydration, fasting glucose, dose of FDG administered, time interval to image acquisition after radiotracer injection) to ensure that the scans are performed under similar circumstances, allowing a meaningful quantitative analysis.

EVALUATION OF ASSOCIATED INFECTIONS BY PET/CT IN PATIENTS WITH SOLID TUMORS

Typically FDG-PET is more sensitive for less differentiated tumors that are greater than 1 cm in size (the threshold for lesion detection is approximately 6 mm, depending on tumor uptake and histology). Well-differentiated tumors, on the contrary, have a lower degree of FDG uptake and occasionally may be a source of false-negative FDG-PET scans.

Posttreatment changes after radiation and chemotherapy can cause increased FDG uptake in both normal and neoplastic tissue, making interpretation of posttherapy scans challenging. Posttreatment images can be further affected by the presence of postsurgical changes, wound healing, and associated infection. Comparison with recent anatomic imaging may be especially helpful and should be performed when available. If a suspicious lesion is present on anatomic imaging, but is not visualized on attenuation-corrected PET images, review of the non–attenuation-corrected images may be useful. Sometimes focal FDG uptake can be less conspicuous or misregistered because of artifacts or patient motion between the time of the transmission scan and subsequent PET image acquisition; this is especially true for lung lesions if the scans are not done with shallow breathing. However, lesions located deep inside the body are generally less conspicuous on the non–attenuation-corrected images than on corrected images.

Postradiation inflammatory reaction accompanied by increased FDG uptake usually subsides sufficiently in 2 to 3 months to allow reevaluation by PET imaging. In some patients, however, significant FDG uptake may persist for up to 6 months after irradiation, significantly complicating interpretation of the PET scan. There are also published reports related to early PET/CT scans performed in patients with non–small-cell lung carcinomas after administration of the first 45 Gy of radiation (ie, approximately 4 weeks after initiation of fractionated radiation therapy, before radiation pneumonitis can develop).[13] The investigators reported a significant correlation in tumor metabolic response on the early and posttherapy PET/CT scans, allowing early changes in the treatment regimens in nonresponders.[13] However, the experience is limited, and larger prospective studies are required to confirm these findings and to evaluate the suitability of early PET/CT scans in routine clinical practice.

In recent years, FDG-PET/CT has been shown to be useful in the assessment of many infectious conditions in patients with malignancy, including postoperative infections such as osteomyelitis, spondylitis, discitis, osteitis, infected metallic implants and hip prostheses in patients with osteosarcoma, infected vascular prosthesis or vascular grafts, septic thrombophlebitis, bacteremia, and opportunistic infection in cancer complicated by AIDS.[1,4,14–21] Thus, focally increased FDG activity in the skeleton should be differentiated from healing fractures, recent wounds, osteomyelitis, and some benign tumors. Acute or healing fractures are normally associated with increased FDG uptake; however, patient history and anatomic imaging can guide interpretation. Postsurgical wounds commonly have moderately increased FDG uptake for up to 2 months, therefore the accuracy of PET can be improved by delaying the imaging during this period. Focal FDG activity adjacent to a joint or joint capsule may mimic a metastatic lesion. Increased FDG activity on the joint surface can also be seen in degenerative disease. Benign tumors such as eosinophilic granulomas, giant cell tumors, and fibrous dysplasia are also FDG avid. Correlation with anatomic images usually reveals the cause of uptake in most cases. Associated increased FDG uptake has been reported in vascular grafts; however, caution must be exercised because this does not necessarily indicate infection. The usefulness of PET/CT in evaluating infectious or inflammatory conditions in patients with the most common solid cancers is described in the following paragraphs.

Restaging head and neck cancers often proves challenging for all imaging modalities because of the altered anatomy after therapy. PET imaging has been reported to have a sensitivity between 80% and 100% in detecting local recurrences.

However, radiation to the head and neck region is frequently accompanied by associated posttreatment changes and increased FDG activity in the epithelium of the oral cavity, pharynx, palatine tonsils, larynx, and paranasal sinuses, decreasing the specificity of FDG-PET. The interpretation can be further complicated by increased FDG uptake in reactive lymph nodes, tense cervical muscles, asymmetric laryngeal muscle activity, or unilateral laryngeal nerve paralysis. The presence of air in the hypermetabolic soft tissue on low-dose CT images is usually suggestive of infection or radiation necrosis. For a better differentiation of FDG activity related to inflammatory and posttreatment changes from residual malignancy, a waiting period of 4 months is usually recommended after radiation therapy to the head and neck region.

For brain tumors, PET can be especially helpful in differentiating posttherapy radiation necrosis from recurrent or residual tumor. The sensitivity of PET in detecting early brain metastases is low because of the high background activity normally present in the brain structures, especially cortex. A flare response has been described in some brain neoplasms, occurring a few days after chemotherapy. It is thought that this temporary increase in FDG activity may be related to a local inflammatory response and increased regional metabolism at the site of massive tumor cell death. Such flare phenomena have been reported in breast cancers after hormonal therapy and certain brain cancers shortly after chemotherapy, and should not be mistaken for progression of hypermetabolic malignancy or lack of response to therapy. In addition, FDG-PET is useful in the diagnosis of brain infections unique to immunocompromised patients. For example, FDG-PET plays an important role in distinguishing central nervous system lymphomas from infections such as toxoplasmosis, and is commonly used for this purpose.[22–24]

In patients with primary lung cancer, PET may be useful in differentiating metabolically active primary tumor from adjacent atelectasis of postobstructive pneumonitis, allowing more accurate preparation of radiation treatment planning. Focal or localized pulmonary parenchymal FDG uptake is usually seen in bacterial pneumonia. In the postoperative period, PET can help differentiate postsurgical scarring and associated reactive changes from recurrent or residual hypermetabolic malignancy. In patients undergoing radiation therapy, however, postradiation pneumonitis is highly FDG avid and may obscure underlying residual malignancy. Detailed knowledge about the position of radiation ports may be of value in certain situations. The inflammatory changes and increased FDG avidity associated with radiation pneumonitis may remain metabolically active on PET imaging for up to 6 months and occasionally even longer. Malignant pleural effusions frequently have low FDG activity caused by dispersion of tumor cells within the fluid, which may render differentiation of malignant from inflammatory effusions challenging or even impossible.

In patients with breast malignancy, FDG-PET is primarily used for evaluation of restaging and response to therapy, although it may be useful occasionally in the evaluation of primary breast lesions. False-negative results may occur in slow-growing tumors, such as tubular and lobular carcinomas, as well as in small lesions such as ductal carcinomas in situ. False-positive results may be caused by inflammatory changes and benign inflammatory processes. Pronounced flare phenomena accompanied by significant increase in FDG uptake can occur in patients with estrogen receptor–positive breast cancers receiving hormonal therapy, especially tamoxifen. In addition, FDG-PET may detect breast tumors incidentally, when the scan is performed for other reasons. Dedicated breast PET imaging systems are being developed (in contrast to whole-body scanners), which may improve not only sensitivity in detecting breast cancers but also differentiation from inflammatory conditions.

THE ROLE OF PET/CT IN EVALUATION OF PATIENTS WITH FEBRILE NEUTROPENIA AND FEVER OF UNKNOWN ORIGIN

Approximately 30% of febrile episodes are subsequently proved to be rooted in infection, as demonstrated by laboratory results or autopsy.[25,26] Clinical diagnosis, however, may be particularly challenging in patients with neutropenia, and conventional imaging frequently fails to reveal the source of fever. FDG-PET has been reported to be a useful modality in the evaluation of fever of unknown origin (FUO) in this situation.[27–31]

Studies have proved that FDG-PET is superior to ^{111}In-labeled white blood cell scan or ^{67}Ga-labeled scintigraphy in identifying the source of fever in patients with febrile neutropenia.[32] Prospective studies in patients with FUO reported that FDG-PET had greater than 80% sensitivity and specificity for identifying the source of fever, exceeding the specificity and sensitivity of gallium scans performed in the same patients.[28] In a study that included 35 patients with FUO, Bleeker-Rovers and colleagues[27] reported 93% sensitivity and 97% specificity for FDG-PET, with a positive predictive value of 87% and a negative predictive value of 95%. In particular, FDG-PET showed promising results in diagnosing infective endo-carditis, which can be a source of FUO in im-munocompromised patients after chemotherapy. Studies performed in such patients showed that despite normal myocardial uptake, FDG-PET can identify sites of infective endocarditis, providing additional information when combined with echo-cardiography.[33] A variety of other conditions, including chronic granulomatous disease, vascu-litis, and even thromboembolic disease, can be the actual cause of FUO and are usually associ-ated with increased FDG uptake.[22,34–36]

In the authors' experience, FDG-PET/CT has proved essential in diagnosing deep-seated mu-cormycosis in a neutropenic patient with FUO as well as in evaluating the subsequent response to antifungal therapy.

EVALUATION OF ASSOCIATED INFECTIONS BY PET/CT IN PATIENTS WITH HEMATOLOGIC MALIGNANCIES

Lymphomas account for almost 8% of all malignancies. Both Hodgkin and non-Hodgkin lymphomas are metabolically active and accumu-late FDG, although the activity may be less pro-nounced in low-grade lymphomas, causing false-negative results. However, an increase in metabolic activity and maximum standardized uptake value in patients with low-grade lym-phomas on follow-up scans is suggestive of transformation to a higher-degree tumor. FDG-PET plays an important role in staging and restag-ing lymphomas, and has been reported to have higher sensitivity (85%–95%) and specificity (up to 95%) than CT for detecting lymphomatous spread to lymph nodes, spleen, and liver. In some patients, PET scans are repeated after 1 or 2 cycles of chemotherapy for response evalua-tion, the results showing good correlation with the ultimate outcome. FDG-PET has also proved superior to ^{67}Ga-labeled single-photon emission CT, which has long been used for staging and re-staging of lymphoma as well as for treatment evaluation. Offering significant advantages such as improved sensitivity, higher resolution, shorter imaging time, and the possibility for quantifica-tion of tracer uptake, PET is gaining increasing support.

In patients with lymphoma, PET can be used to evaluate bone marrow involvement, although caution must be exercised in patients who have received chemotherapy or colony-growth stimu-lating factor as part of their treatment, because the reactive bone marrow activity in such cases can frequently produce increased FDG uptake throughout the skeleton. This activity is generally nonfocal and can persist for 2 to 3 weeks after chemotherapy. The pattern is easily differentiated from metastatic disease in most patients; how-ever, excessive background activity occasionally can mask the actual lesions and local tumor involvement. Waiting for a period of 2 to 4 weeks after chemotherapy is usually sufficient to avoid interfering bone marrow activity. Increased FDG uptake in the thymus after lymphoma therapy is known as thymic rebound. The characteristic shape of the activity resembling the thymus in the anterior mediastinum can serve as a diagnostic clue, although intense activity may be difficult to differentiate from tumor involvement in some patients.

Low-grade non-Hodgkin lymphomas, such as follicular lymphoma, small-cell lymphocytic lymphoma, and mucosa-associated lymphoma tissue, are less FDG avid, and can cause false-negative results or complicate interpretation. False-positive results have also been reported and can be caused by concurrent inflammation or infection, including osteomyelitis, infected pros-theses, fungal and granulomatous diseases, and even infectious mononucleosis.[37–41] Increased FDG activity in the right lower quadrant in a patient with treated lymphoma is shown in **Fig. 1**. The uptake proved to be due to appendicitis and the patient subsequently underwent surgery.

Hypermetabolic activity in the spleen visualized on PET/CT scans in patients with lymphoma has been associated not only with lymphoma infiltra-tion but also with local infections such as *Toxo-plasma gondii*.[42] Frequently, however, increased splenic activity in patients with infection may represent increased glucose use by the spleen, which is an integral part of the body's immune system. Therefore the uptake cannot be automat-ically attributed to infection or tumor infiltration, and further investigations are warranted if clinically indicated.[22]

In patients with leukemia, PET/CT may be useful in detecting extramedullary involvement; however, studies in this area are limited.[43–45] The modality has already proved its value in diagnosing Richter transformation of chronic lymphoid leukemia to diffuse large-cell lymphoma, with a reported 91% sensitivity and 80% specificity.[46] In addition, PET/CT can be a valuable tool in diagnosing a variety of infectious and inflammatory conditions in patients with leukemia, similar to those described in FUO. Previously the authors reported their experience in detecting fungal infection on PET/CT scans in patients with leukemia with disseminated candidiasis.[47] The modality also proved useful in evaluating the therapeutic response to antifungal therapy, with all patients

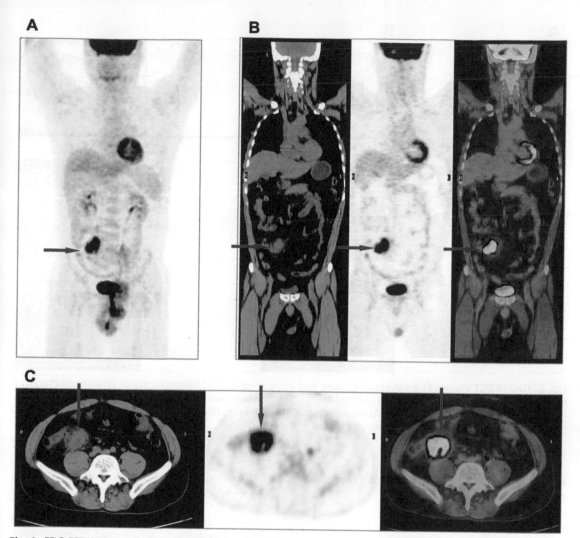

Fig. 1. FDG-PET/CT images of a patient with natural killer/T-cell lymphoma (nasal type), status post chemotherapy and radiation therapy 2 years ago. Despite no abnormal FDG activity in the nasal cavity at the site of known lymphoma, unexpected focal FDG uptake was detected in the right lower quadrant (*arrow*). The patient proved to have appendicitis, subsequently confirmed during surgical intervention and on biopsy of the excised appendix. (*A*) Maximum-intensity projection (MIP) image; (*B*) coronal image; (*C*) transaxial image.

achieving favorable outcomes. The PET/CT images of a patient with acute myeloblastic leukemia and disseminated candidiasis are shown in **Fig. 2**.

Mahfouz and colleagues[48] found that FDG-PET is a useful tool in the management of infection in patients with multiple myeloma. In their investigation, medical records of 248 patients with multiple myeloma who had FDG-PET scans were reviewed. The investigators found 165 episodes of infection in 143 patients. Among these episodes, 46 were identified only by FDG-PET and not by any other modalities. In addition, FDG-PET detected 20 silent but clinically relevant episodes of infection. Moreover, the findings of FDG-PET led

to a change in the further management of 55 episodes of infection. Mahfouz and colleagues[48] concluded that FDG-PET is a useful tool in this clinical setting, even instances of severe immunosuppression. Routine use of FDG-PET/CT in high-risk patients has resulted in not only lower morbidity and mortality[20] but also improved cost-effectiveness.[49]

In summary, FDG-PET/CT is not only an established imaging modality for diagnosing and staging malignancies but is also a valuable tool for detecting associated infections in oncology patients. However, the published reports on this topic in the world literature are limited, and new developments are required to further define the roles of

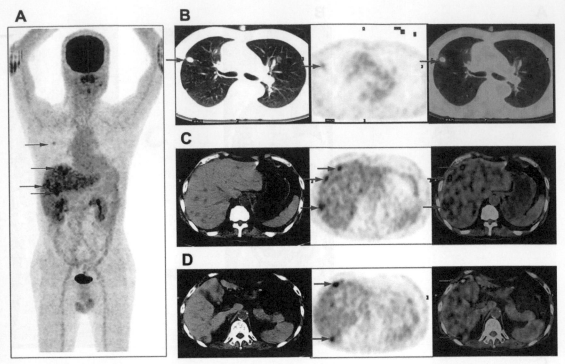

Fig. 2. FDG-PET/CT images of a patient with fever and acute myeloblastic leukemia, status post chemotherapy 5 months ago. Multiple FDG-avid lesions (*arrows*) are noted in the liver and right lung, representing chronic disseminated candidiasis confirmed by microbiological tests. (*A*) MIP image; (*B*) transaxial image showing lung lesions; (*C* and *D*) transaxial image showing hepatic lesions.

FDG-PET/CT in the management of infections in patients with malignancies.

REFERENCES

1. Bleeker-Rovers CP, Vos FJ, van der Graaf WT, et al. Nuclear medicine imaging of infection in cancer patients (with emphasis on FDG-PET). Oncologist 2011;16:980–91.
2. Wisplinghoff H, Cornely OA, Moser S, et al. Outcomes of nosocomial bloodstream infections in adult neutropenic patients: a prospective cohort and matched case-control study. Infect Control Hosp Epidemiol 2003;24(12):905–11.
3. Worth LJ, Seymour JF, Slavin MA. Infective and thrombotic complications of central venous catheters in patients with hematological malignancy: prospective evaluation of nontunneled devices. Support Care Cancer 2009;17(7):811–8.
4. Wong PS, Lau WE, Worth LJ, et al. Clinically important detection of infection as an 'incidental' finding during cancer staging using FDG-PET/CT. Intern Med J 2011. [Epub ahead of print].
5. Yang Y, Fang Hua. [Nosocomial infection in cancer patients during chemotherapy: a clinical analysis].
   Chinese Journal of Nosocomiology 2003;13(7): 638–9 [in Chinese].
6. Worth LJ, Slavin MA, Brown GV, et al. Catheter-related bloodstream infections in hematology: time for standardized surveillance? Cancer 2007; 109(7):1215–26.
7. Almuhaideb A, Papathanasiou N, Bomanji J. ^{18}F-FDG PET/CT imaging in oncology. Ann Saudi Med 2011;31:3–13.
8. Barrington SF, O'Doherty MJ. Limitations of PET for imaging lymphoma. Eur J Nucl Med Mol Imaging 2003;30:S117–27.
9. Cheng G, Chen W, Chamroonrat W, et al. Biopsy versus FDG PET/CT in the initial evaluation of bone marrow involvement in pediatric lymphoma patients. Eur J Nucl Med Mol Imaging 1469;38:1469–76.
10. Houseni M, Chamroonrat W, Zhuang J, et al. Prognostic implication of dual-phase PET in adenocarcinoma of the lung. J Nucl Med 2010;51: 535–42.
11. Anderson GS, Brinkmann F, Soulen MC, et al. FDG positron emission tomography in the surveillance of hepatic tumors treated with radiofrequency ablation. Clin Nucl Med 2003;28:192–7.
12. de Winter F, van de Wiele C, Vogelaers D, et al. Fluorine-18 fluorodeoxyglucose-position emission

tomography: a highly accurate imaging modality for the diagnosis of chronic musculoskeletal infections. J Bone Joint Surg Am 2001;83:651–60.

13. Kong FM, Frey KA, Quint LE, et al. A pilot study of [18F]fluorodeoxyglucose positron emission tomography scans during and after radiation-based therapy in patients with non small-cell lung cancer. J Clin Oncol 2007;25:3116–23.

14. Miceli M, Atoui R, Walker R, et al. Diagnosis of deep septic thrombophlebitis in cancer patients by fluorine-18 fluorodeoxyglucose positron emission tomography scanning: a preliminary report. J Clin Oncol 2004;22:1949–56.

15. Wan DQ, Joseph UA, Barron BJ, et al. Ventriculoperitoneal shunt catheter and cerebral spinal fluid infection initially detected by FDG PET/CT scan. Clin Nucl Med 2009;34:464–5.

16. Zhuang H, Chacko TK, Hickeson M, et al. Persistent non-specific FDG uptake on PET imaging following hip arthroplasty. Eur J Nucl Med Mol Imaging 2002;29:1328–33.

17. Chacko TK, Zhuang H, Nakhoda KZ, et al. Applications of fluorodeoxyglucose positron emission tomography in the diagnosis of infection. Nucl Med Commun 2003;24:615–24.

18. Keidar Z, Engel A, Hoffman A, et al. Prosthetic vascular graft infection: the role of 18F-FDG PET/CT. J Nucl Med 2007;48:1230–6.

19. Santiago JF, Jana S, Gilbert HM, et al. Role of fluorine-18-fluorodeoxyglucose in the work-up of febrile AIDS patients: experience with dual head coincidence imaging. Clin Positron Imaging 1999;2:301–9.

20. Vos FJ, Bleeker-Rovers CP, Sturm PD, et al. 18F-FDG PET/CT for detection of metastatic infection in gram-positive bacteremia. J Nucl Med 2010;51:1234–40.

21. Imperiale A, Federici L, Lefebvre N, et al. F-18 FDG PET/CT as a valuable imaging tool for assessing treatment efficacy in inflammatory and infectious diseases. Clin Nucl Med 2010;35:86–90.

22. Love C, Tomas MB, Tronco GG, et al. FDG PET of infection and inflammation. Radiographics 2005;25:1357–68.

23. Hoffman JM, Waskin HA, Schifter T, et al. FDG-PET in differentiating lymphoma from nonmalignant central nervous system lesions in patients with AIDS. J Nucl Med 1993;34:567–75.

24. O'Doherty MJ, Barrington SF, Campbell M, et al. PET scanning and the human immunodeficiency virus-positive patient. J Nucl Med 1997;38:1575–83.

25. Efstathiou SP, Pefanis AV, Tsiakou AG, et al. Fever of unknown origin: discrimination between infectious and non-infectious causes. Eur J Intern Med 2010;21:137–43.

26. Roongpoovapatr P, Suankratay C. Causative pathogens of fever in neutropenic patients at King Chulalongkorn Memorial Hospital. J Med Assoc Thai 2010;93:776–83.

27. Bleeker-Rovers CP, de Kleijn EM, Corstens FH, et al. Clinical value of FDG PET in patients with fever of unknown origin and patients suspected of focal infection or inflammation. Eur J Nucl Med Mol Imaging 2004;31:29–37.

28. Meller J, Altenvoerde G, Munzel U, et al. Fever of unknown origin: prospective comparison of [18F] FDG imaging with a double-head coincidence camera and gallium-67 citrate SPET. Eur J Nucl Med 2000;27:1617–25.

29. Blockmans D, Knockaert D, Maes A, et al. Clinical value of [(18)F]fluoro-deoxyglucose positron emission tomography for patients with fever of unknown origin. Clin Infect Dis 2001;32:191–6.

30. Lorenzen J, Buchert R, Bohuslavizki KH. Value of FDG PET in patients with fever of unknown origin. Nucl Med Commun 2001;22:779–83.

31. Simons KS, Pickkers P, Bleeker-Rovers CP, et al. F-18-fluorodeoxyglucose positron emission tomography combined with CT in critically ill patients with suspected infection. Intensive Care Med 2009;36:504–11.

32. Ferda J, Ferdová E, Zahlava J, et al. Fever of unknown origin: a value of 18F-FDG-PET/CT with integrated full diagnostic isotropic CT imaging. Eur J Radiol 2010;73:518–25.

33. Yen RF, Chen YC, Wu YW, et al. Using 18-fluoro-2-deoxyglucose positron emission tomography in detecting infectious endocarditis/endoarteritis: a preliminary report. Acad Radiol 2004;11:316–21.

34. Blockmans D, Stroobants S, Maes A, et al. Positron emission tomography in giant cell arteritis and polymyalgia rheumatica: evidence for inflammation of the aortic arch. Am J Med 2000;108:246–9.

35. Bleeker-Rovers CP, Bredie SJ, van der Meer JW, et al. Fluorine 18 fluorodeoxyglucose positron emission tomography in the diagnosis and follow-up of three patients with vasculitis. Am J Med 2004;116:50–3.

36. Meller J, Strutz F, Siefker U, et al. Early diagnosis and follow-up of aortitis with [(18)F]FDG PET and MRI. Eur J Nucl Med Mol Imaging 2003;30:730–6.

37. Guhlmann A, Brecht-Krauss D, Suger G, et al. Fluorine-18-FDG PET and technetium-99m antigranulocyte antibody scintigraphy in chronic osteomyelitis. J Nucl Med 1998;39:2145–52.

38. Toshihide K, Yoshichika S, Syunji T, et al. Pulmonary intravascular lymphoma complicated with Pneumocystis carinii pneumonia: a case report. Jpn J Clin Oncol 2001;31(7):333–6.

39. Romsee GM, Mortelmans L. PET versus PET-CT in patient with suspicion of non-Hodgkin lymphoma recurrence. Clin Nucl Med 2007;32:954–5.

40. Lustberg MB, Aras O, Meisenberg BR, et al. FDG PET/CT findings in acute adult mononucleosis mimicking malignant lymphoma. Eur J Haematol 2008;81(2):154–6.

41. Zhuang H, Alavi A. 18-Fluorodeoxyglucose positron emission tomographic imaging in the detection and monitoring of infection and inflammation. Semin Nucl Med 2002;32:47–59.

42. Sandherr M, von Schilling C, Link T, et al. Pitfalls in imaging Hodgkin's disease with computed tomography and positron emission tomography using fluorine-18-fluorodeoxyglucose. Ann Oncol 2001;12:719–22.

43. Karlin L, Itti E, Pautas C, et al. PET-imaging as a useful tool for early detection of the relapse site in the management of primary myeloid sarcoma. Haematologica 2006;91:E148–9.

44. Kuenzle K, Taverna C, Steinert HC. Detection of extramedullary infiltrates in acute myelogenous leukemia with whole-body positron emission tomography and 2-deoxy-2-^{18}F-fluoro-D-glucose. Mol Imaging Biol 2002;4:179–83.

45. von Falck C, Laenger F, Knapp WH, et al. F-18 FDG PET/CT showing bilateral breast involvement in acute myeloid leukemia relapse. Clin Nucl Med 2009;34:713–5.

46. Bruzzi JF, Macapinlac H, Tsimberidou AM, et al. Detection of Richter's transformation of chronic lymphocytic leukemia by PET/CT. J Nucl Med 2006;47:1267–73.

47. Xu B, Shi P, Wu H, et al. Utility of FDG PET/CT in guiding antifungal therapy in acute leukemia patients with chronic disseminated candidiasis. Clin Nucl Med 2010;35:567–70.

48. Mahfouz T, Miceli MH, Saghafifar F, et al. ^{18}F-fluorodeoxyglucose positron emission tomography contributes to the diagnosis and management of infections in patients with multiple myeloma: a study of 165 infectious episodes. J Clin Oncol 2005;23:7857–63.

49. Vos FJ, Bleeker-Rovers CP, Kullberg BJ, et al. Cost-effectiveness of routine (18)F-FDG PET/CT in high-risk patients with gram-positive bacteremia. J Nucl Med 2011;52:1673–8.

The Utility of FDG PET/CT in Inflammatory Bowel Disease

Roland Hustinx, MD, PhD

KEYWORDS

- PET/CT • Crohn disease • Ulcerative colitis
- Inflammatory bowel disease

Inflammatory bowel diseases (IBD) are chronic immune-mediated inflammatory diseases that affect the gastrointestinal tract. Two distinct entities are recognized: Crohn disease (CD) and ulcerative colitis (UC). The pathophysiologic processes behind IBD are complex and an excellent review has been published by Khor and colleagues.[1] It may be summarized as an inappropriate and continuing inflammatory response to commensal microbes in a generically susceptible host.[1] Pathologic changes observed in CD include transmural inflammation, which is limited to the mucosa and submucosa in UC. CD may affect any part of the digestive tract, although the terminal ileum and perianal regions are the most frequent locations. UC is limited to the colon, starting in the rectum and progressing proximally toward the cecum. Both entities are chronic relapsing diseases, but their clinical evolution is different. In UC, periods of activity and remission are often well delineated, whereas CD is more often a chronic active disease with a continuous inflammatory process. UC is usually not associated with the development of intestinal complications, probably due to its essentially mucosal inflammation. In contrast, CD is frequently complicated by fibrotic and/or deeply penetrating lesions leading to intestinal strictures and/or fistulas. These complications affect a few patients at the time of diagnosis but can be present in up to 50% to 60% of patients after 10 years of evolution.[2]

Therapeutic strategies for IBD changed greatly with the introduction of infliximab, the first anti–tumor necrosis factor (TNF) agent, in 1998. The available medications include aminosalicylates, corticosteroids, thiopurines, methotrexate, and anti-TNF agents. In mild to moderate UC, 5-aminosalicylates are the first choice, either orally or locally (enemas or suppositories). In cases of inadequate response after 2 to 4 weeks, steroids are given in combination with 5-aminosalicylates. Patients who become steroid dependent receive thiopurines. Refractory UC is defined as an active disease despite steroids or a disease that does not respond to thiopurines. Those patients are given anti-TNF drugs with objective response rates ranging from 55% to 78%.[3] The strategy is similar in CD, except that 5-aminosalicylates are less effective and tend to be replaced by budesonide, a glucocorticoid steroid, as the first-line drug. Other differences include a greater role for immunomodulators such as methotrexate and a more frequent need for surgery.[3] Major questions arise on the timing for switching from one treatment to another and the duration of the treatment. No drug permanently modifies the pattern of IBD progression. High relapse rates are observed after withdrawal of therapy. As a result, if the treatment is efficient and well tolerated, it is usually maintained. The issue of the end point also remains unsettled. A recent meta-analysis has shown that anti-TNF drugs are effective for inducing short-term response, maintaining long-term clinical relief, and reducing the colectomy rate in UC. However, they fail to improve the quality of life and the mucosal healing.[4] The current clinical management of IBD is hampered by the absence of objective measures of disease activity

Division of Nuclear Medicine, University Hospital of Liège, University of Liège, B-4000 Liège, Belgium
E-mail address: rhustinx@chu.ulg.ac.be

PET Clin 7 (2012) 219–225
doi:10.1016/j.cpet.2012.01.009
1556-8598/12/$ – see front matter © 2012 Elsevier Inc. All rights reserved

and predictors of evolution. Conventional clinical scales such as the Crohn Disease Activity Index (CDAI) include subjective parameters that limit their value. Biomarkers such as fecal calprotectin or serum C-reactive protein (CRP) may be helpful for monitoring the disease, but none offers a reliable estimation of the pattern of disease development and evolution.[5] The analogy with rheumatoid arthritis (RA) is tempting because both IBD and RA are immune-mediated inflammatory diseases in which anti-TNF drugs play an important role. It has been shown in RA that the early introduction of anti-TNF drugs prevents structural joint damage and long-term morbidity. There is currently limited evidence that this principle might be extended to IBD, largely because of the imperfections of the currently available tools for assessing the activity of the disease. Innovative approaches that include both cross-sectional imaging and endoscopic imaging are being proposed,[6] and metabolic imaging may play a crucial role in this task.

FLUORODEOXYGLUCOSE-PET IMAGING

The initial suggestion that fluorodeoxyglucose (FDG)-PET might be used for assessing activity of IBD came in the form of a letter to the *Lancet* as early as 1997.[7] In 6 patients, and with nonattenuation corrected PET, Bicik and colleagues[7] were able to show a correlation between FDG uptake, endoscopic anomalies, or histologic evidence of inflammation in areas that were endoscopically normal. Skehan and colleagues[8] described the use of FDG-PET in a pediatric population of 25 patients including 15 with CD, 3 with UC, and 7 with nonspecific abdominal pain or diarrhea. The sensitivity was 81% and the specificity 85% for identifying patients with IBD. Similar results were obtained by the same group in a larger series of 65 children, including 37 with newly diagnosed IBD.[9] Neurath and colleagues[10] studied 59 patients with CD. Comparing FDG-PET, hydro–magnetic resonance imaging, and granulocyte antibodies scintigraphy, all 3 techniques had a high specificity but FDG-PET was the most sensitive method in the subgroup of patients with endoscopic verification. The investigators found visual analysis of the PET images to be most accurate, because the standardized uptake values (SUVs) were not correlated with any of the other indicators of CD activity, such as the CDAI, CRP levels, or inflamed segments visualized at colonoscopy. In contrast, other investigators reported sensitivity of 98%, a specificity of 68%, and an accuracy of 83% using a cutoff of 1.2 for the target lesion maximal SUV (SUVmax)/liver SUV ratio.[11]

However, the series was limited (23 patients), retrospective, and heterogeneous.

FDG-PET/COMPUTED TOMOGRAPHY

The high sensitivity of FDG PET for detecting active IBD is expected, but specificity remains an issue because bowel uptake, which is sometimes high, is frequently observed in the absence of any disease.[12] In contrast, when focal metabolic abnormalities are matched with abnormal soft tissue density or wall thickening on PET/computed tomography (CT), they most often correspond with disease, whether these are inflammatory or tumoral lesions.[13] The first report on the use of PET/CT in IBD was published by Louis and colleagues[14] in 2007. FDG-PET/CT and ileocolonoscopy were obtained within 1 week in 22 patients with CD and a clinical or biological suspicion of active disease. The CDAI was calculated, and serum CRP and fecal calprotectin were measured before endoscopy. The Crohn Disease Endoscopy Index of Severity (CDEIS) was also recorded. Overall, the sensitivity for detecting all endoscopic lesions was 72.9% (35 of 48 endoscopically affected segments). Most importantly, PET/CT detected all the severe endoscopic lesions (14/14 deep ulcers and strictures). The global PET/CT score significantly correlated with the endoscopic score (CDEIS), clinical score (CDAI), and biological findings (CRP). A receiver operating characteristic (ROC) analysis showed that the optimal cutoff for the lesion/liver SUV ratio was 1.47. Using this cutoff, the sensitivity for detecting severe endoscopic lesions was 100% and the specificity was 67%. CT was mostly useful for accurately localizing the areas of increased uptake, but the logistic regression analysis showed that, unlike the SUV, bowel wall thickening was not independently associated with the presence of severe lesions. However, the CT did not take full advantage of the diagnostic capabilities of the technique. Water was used as an oral contrast agent, no intravenous iodinated contrast was given, and the acquisition parameters (slice thickness, 2.5 mm; pitch, 1.5; table feed, 15 mm/s; 120 kV; 50 mA s) were set to minimize the patient's irradiation. As discussed later, the contribution of CT imaging can go further than in the aforementioned study. A similar correlation between disease activity and PET/low-dose CT findings was reported in 12 patients with IBD, including 7 with CD and 5 with UC.[15] Two examples of active CD are shown in **Figs. 1** and **2**.

As mentioned earlier, surgery may be needed in CD, especially in patients with obstructive symptoms. Such symptoms may be related to intestinal wall muscle hypertrophy and fibrotic stenosis or

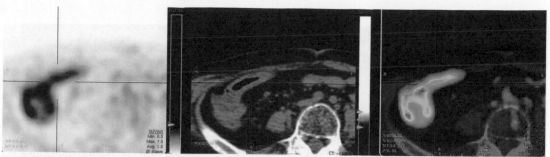

Fig. 1. A 68-year-old woman with a long-standing history of CD treated with mesalamine. FDG-PET/CT is performed to evaluate clinical degradation. It shows increased uptake in the terminal ileum and ileocolic junction. Budesonide was introduced, with a good clinical response.

acute transmural inflammation. The distinction is relevant because acute transmural inflammation is better managed using medical treatment than surgery. Jacene and colleagues[16] performed FDG-PET/CT in 13 patients who were scheduled for surgery in this setting. There was no correlation between FDG uptake, assessed visually or using the SUV normalized for lean body mass (SUL), and any of the clinical and laboratory parameters of inflammation. There was also no correlation between FDG uptake and the pathologic pattern (ie, fibrosis or hypertrophy and inflammation). An ROC analysis identified a cutoff value of 8 for the SUL as the best for detecting active inflammation in the bowel, albeit with a sensitivity of 60% and a specificity of 100%.

Little is known regarding FDG-PET/CT in treatment monitoring, although this is likely to be the most important indication if the technique is to enter routine clinical practice (**Fig. 3**). The evolution of the metabolic activity on FDG-PET/CT was correlated with the clinical improvements described after treatment with steroids or infliximab in a series of 5 patients.[17] The potential of FDG-PET for quantitatively assessing bowel inflammation was elegantly shown by Brewer and colleagues[18] in a series of animal experiments. Using microPET and microCT in a murine model of colitis, they were first able to show that FDG uptake in the inflamed bowel wall was associated with glucose transporter 1 levels in mucosal CD4(+) T lymphocytes but not other intestinal immune cell types. This increased uptake appears early in the disease process, so microPET measurements were positive at the stage of preclinical inflammation. Furthermore, when intestinal inflammation was increased by treatment with piroxicam and decreased with anti-TL1A treatment, FDG uptake was correspondingly altered. Extended to the human setting, such findings would provide the basis for a reliable noninvasive assessment of bowel wall inflammation during treatment.

PET/CT Enterography

CT enterography (CTe) detects ileal inflammation related to CD with a sensitivity ranging from 75% to 90%.[19] For the colon, the sensitivity is 74%.[20] Enteric neutral contrast agents are given to the patients to distend the lumen of the bowel. In

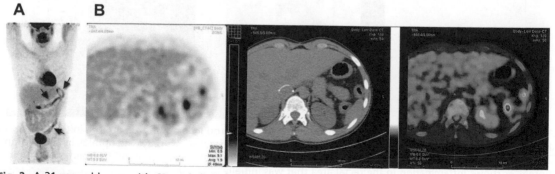

Fig. 2. A 21-year-old man with CD and clinical signs of evolution. PET shows increased uptake in the transverse and descending colon, shown by the arrows on the three-dimensional projection image (A). The corresponding transverse sections (B) show bowel thickening, although caution should be applied when reading such low-dose, unprepared, CT scans.

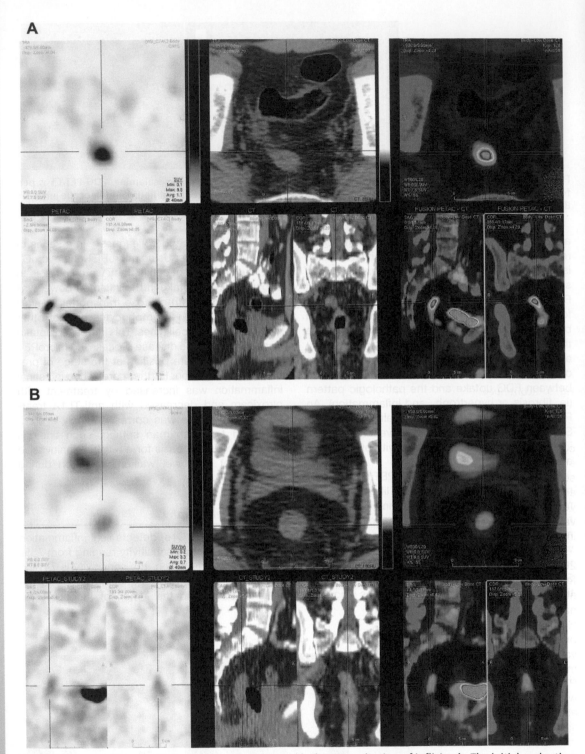

Fig. 3. A 32-year-old man with known CD is investigated before introduction of infliximab. The initial evaluation shows highly increased rectal uptake (*A*). Further evaluation 1 year later shows only mild uptake, in line with the clinical improvement (*B*). Because of fever of unknown origin, infliximab is withdrawn. PET/CT performed rapidly thereafter shows inflammation in the rectal area that was initially affected (*C*).

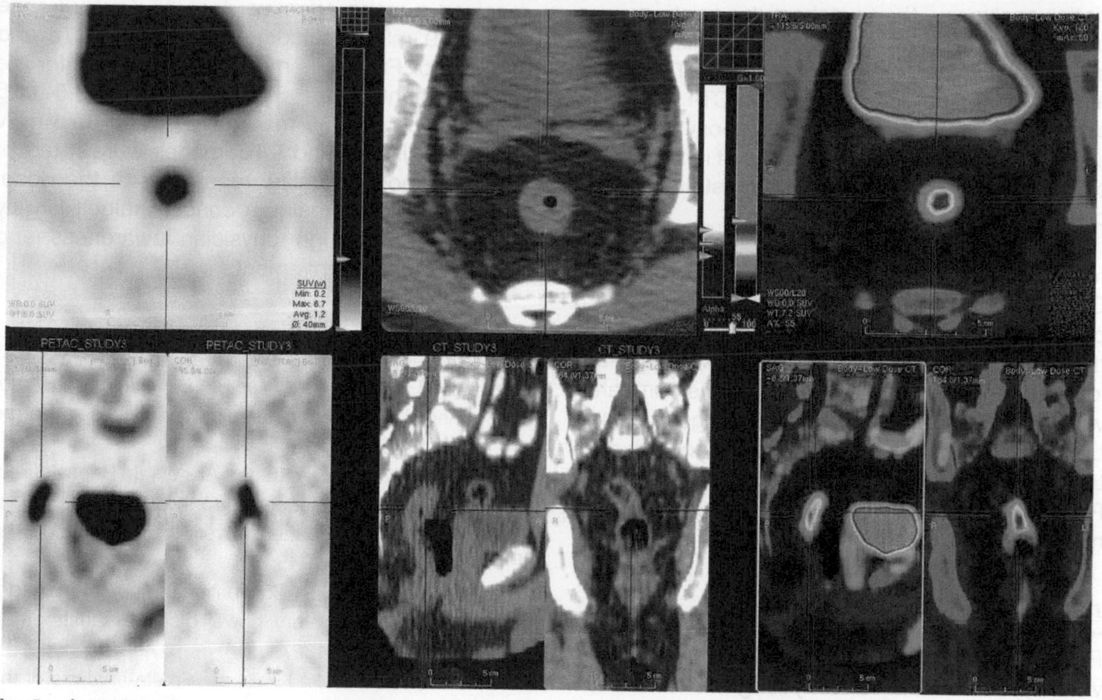

Fig. 3. (*continued*)

combination with intravenous iodinated contrast enhancement, changes in the inflamed bowel segments can be visualized, such as mural enhancement or increased thickness. In recent years, several studies evaluated the diagnostic value of combining PET and CTe in a single imaging procedure.

Groshar and colleagues[21] performed PET/CTe in 28 patients with known or suspected CD. They found significant correlations between the CT abnormalities, such as mural thickness and enhancement, and the metabolic activity (SUVmax). However, they did not study the clinical, biological, or endoscopic parameters, and the clinical relevance of such observations remains unknown. Ahmadi and colleagues[22] retrospectively reviewed 41 PET/CTe scans in patients with CD. The analysis was completed for the 30 patients who showed abnormal imaging results. A total of 48 bowel segments were identified on CTe, among which 38 (79%) showed abnormal FDG uptake. There was no instance of abnormal segment on PET that did not show any abnormality on CTe. The only positive finding was that the presence of mucosal enhancement without increased FDG uptake was associated with failure of medical therapy. There was no correlation between the metabolic activity and any of the clinical or biological scores of inflammation. With CTe, there was only a weak correlation with the erythrocyte sedimentation rate and none with the other biological and clinical parameters. Because endoscopy was not performed, the gold standard for identifying inflammation is weak. In addition, the study is limited by several methodological weaknesses: enhanced CT was used for generating the attenuation-corrected PET images. Although this does not reduce the image quality, this may affect the quantitative measurements (SUVs). Such bias might not be considered clinically significant but it should be evaluated in an appropriate fashion. In addition, several investigators reported strong correlations with endoscopic and clinical parameters of inflammation using activity ratios rather than the absolute SUVmax.[10,11,14]

Shyn and colleagues[23] compared PET/CTe with CTe alone in 13 patients with CD. In this study, comparisons were made with clinical and endoscopic scores. All bowel segments with more than mild inflammation were identified by visual interpretation of PET/CTe and CTe, with a specificity of 89.7%. A significant correlation was found between the pathologic inflammation grade and both the metabolic activity and the CTe score. In the patient-based analysis, the SUV ratio showed the strongest correlation, whereas, in the segment-based analysis, it was the CTe score. In both analyses, the weakest correlation was observed using the SUVmax. In contrast with the study by Ahmadi and colleagues,[22] PET revealed additional findings compared with CTe in 3 of 13 cases. There were 2 cases of positive bowel segment on PET without evidence of inflammation on CTe, and 1 case of enterocolic fistula not seen on CTe.

Das and colleagues[24] proposed PET/CT colonography and PET/CT enteroclysis[25] in UC and CD, respectively. There was a good correlation between the combined imaging techniques and the endoscopic score in CD, whereas PET/CT colonography detected additional lesions compared with colonoscopy in UC. These findings remain to be confirmed by other investigators, and the relative role of these techniques, compared with PET/low-dose CT, or PET/CTe, is likely to remain marginal.

Dosimetry

Radiation dose is of particular concern in IBDs, which predominantly affect young adults. Furthermore, IBDs are chronic ailments that require multiple explorations throughout the patients' lifetime. In a series of 103 patients with CD diagnosed between 1990 and 2001 and followed up for an average of 8.9 years, the median total effective dose was 26.6 mSv ranging from 0 to 279 mSV.[26] CT examinations contributed to half of the total effective dose. A diagnosis of CD made during childhood and severe disease are associated with a higher cumulative exposure.[27]

The acquisition parameters used in the study by Louis and colleagues[14] led to a radiation dose per procedure that is largely acceptable in an adult population. Using the most recent PET/CT scanners, exposure may be further reduced by decreasing the injected dose at the expense of a slight increase in acquisition time to maintain the counting statistics. When the recommended doses of FDG are used in children, the effective dose from the PET procedure varies from 5 mSv in 1-year-old infants to 8.6 mSv in adolescents.[28] Considering the CT procedure, low-dose CT may decrease the exposure by a factor of 2 compared with a diagnostic CT. Furthermore, it is possible that, in the setting of IBD, a low-dose CT, mainly used for attenuation correction, would be sufficient for clinical efficacy. Such low-exposure CT may decrease the radiation dose to 3% of the level resulting from a conventional CT study. However, recent data suggest an added value for combined PET and CTe studies.[21,23] Shyn and colleagues[20] adapted their acquisition protocol in the course

of their prospective study. The first 4 patients received a mean effective dose 17.7 mSv (range 13.9–23.9 mSv), including 7.7 mSv for CTe and 10 mSv for FDG. The mean effective dose for the other patients was 8.3 mSv (range 6.5–11.5 mSv), including 4.56 mSv for CTe and 3.75 mSv for FDG. All PET and CTe images were rated of good diagnostic quality, regardless of the dose. Radiation dose remains a concern, albeit largely manageable through physician awareness and technological improvements.

REFERENCES

1. Khor B, Gardet A, Xavier RJ. Genetics and pathogenesis of inflammatory bowel disease. Nature 2011;474:307.
2. Louis E, Collard A, Oger AF, et al. Behaviour of Crohn's disease according to the Vienna classification: changing pattern over the course of the disease. Gut 2001;49:777.
3. Burger D, Travis S. Conventional medical management of inflammatory bowel disease. Gastroenterology 2011;140:1827.
4. Huang X, Lv B, Jin HF, et al. A meta-analysis of the therapeutic effects of tumor necrosis factor-alpha blockers on ulcerative colitis. Eur J Clin Pharmacol 2011;67:759.
5. Lewis JD. The utility of biomarkers in the diagnosis and therapy of inflammatory bowel disease. Gastroenterology 2011;140:1817.
6. Pariente B, Cosnes J, Danese S, et al. Development of the Crohn's disease digestive damage score, the Lemann score. Inflamm Bowel Dis 2011;17:1415.
7. Bicik I, Bauerfeind P, Breitbach T, et al. Inflammatory bowel disease activity measured by positron-emission tomography. Lancet 1997;350:262.
8. Skehan SJ, Issenman R, Mernagh J, et al. 18F-Fluorodeoxyglucose positron tomography in diagnosis of paediatric inflammatory bowel disease. Lancet 1999;354:836.
9. Lemberg DA, Issenman RM, Cawdron R, et al. Positron emission tomography in the investigation of pediatric inflammatory bowel disease. Inflamm Bowel Dis 2005;11:733.
10. Neurath MF, Vehling D, Schunk K, et al. Noninvasive assessment of Crohn's disease activity: a comparison of 18F-fluorodeoxyglucose positron emission tomography, hydromagnetic resonance imaging, and granulocyte scintigraphy with labeled antibodies. Am J Gastroenterol 2002;97:1978.
11. Loffler M, Weckesser M, Franzius C, et al. High diagnostic value of 18F-FDG-PET in pediatric patients with chronic inflammatory bowel disease. Ann N Y Acad Sci 2006;1072:379.
12. Cook GJ, Maisey MN, Fogelman I, Normal variants, artefacts and interpretative pitfalls in PET imaging

with 18-fluoro-2-deoxyglucose and carbon-11 methionine. Eur J Nucl Med 1999;26:1363.

13. Kamel EM, Thumshirn M, Truninger K, et al. Significance of incidental 18F-FDG accumulations in the gastrointestinal tract in PET/CT: correlation with endoscopic and histopathologic results. J Nucl Med 2004;45:1804.

14. Louis E, Ancion G, Colard A, et al. Noninvasive assessment of Crohn's disease intestinal lesions with (18)F-FDG PET/CT. J Nucl Med 2007;48:1053.

15. Meisner RS, Spier BJ, Einarsson S, et al. Pilot study using PET/CT as a novel, noninvasive assessment of disease activity in inflammatory bowel disease. Inflamm Bowel Dis 2007;13:993.

16. Jacene HA, Ginsburg P, Kwon J, et al. Prediction of the need for surgical intervention in obstructive Crohn's disease by 18F-FDG PET/CT. J Nucl Med 2009;50:1751.

17. Spier BJ, Perlman SB, Jaskowiak CJ, et al. PET/CT in the evaluation of inflammatory bowel disease: studies in patients before and after treatment. Mol Imaging Biol 2009;12:85.

18. Brewer S, McPherson M, Fujiwara D, et al. Molecular imaging of murine intestinal inflammation with 2-deoxy-2-[18F]fluoro-D-glucose and positron emission tomography. Gastroenterology 2008;135:744.

19. Fletcher JG, Fidler JL, Bruining DH, et al. New concepts in intestinal imaging for inflammatory bowel diseases. Gastroenterology 2011;140:1795.

20. Johnson KT, Hara AK, Johnson CD. Evaluation of colitis: usefulness of CT enterography technique. Emerg Radiol 2009;16:277.

21. Groshar D, Bernstine H, Stern D, et al. PET/CT enterography in Crohn disease: correlation of disease activity on CT enterography with 18F-FDG uptake. J Nucl Med 2010;51:1009.

22. Ahmadi A, Li Q, Muller K, et al. Diagnostic value of noninvasive combined fluorine-18 labeled fluoro-2-deoxy-D-glucose positron emission tomography and computed tomography enterography in active Crohn's disease. Inflamm Bowel Dis 2010;16:974.

23. Shyn PB, Mortele KJ, Britz-Cunningham SH, et al. Low-dose 18F-FDG PET/CT enterography: improving on CT enterography assessment of patients with Crohn disease. J Nucl Med 2010;51:1841.

24. Das CJ, Makharia GK, Kumar R, et al. PET/CT colonography: a novel non-invasive technique for assessment of extent and activity of ulcerative colitis. Eur J Nucl Med Mol Imaging 2010;37:714.

25. Das CJ, Makharia G, Kumar R, et al. PET-CT enteroclysis: a new technique for evaluation of inflammatory diseases of the intestine. Eur J Nucl Med Mol Imaging 2007;34:2106.

26. Peloquin JM, Pardi DS, Sandborn WJ, et al. Diagnostic ionizing radiation exposure in a population-based cohort of patients with inflammatory bowel disease. Am J Gastroenterol 2008;103:2015.

27. Desmond AN, O'Regan K, Curran C, et al. Crohn's disease: factors associated with exposure to high levels of diagnostic radiation. Gut 2008;57:1524.

28. Gelfand MJ, Lemen LC. PET/CT and SPECT/CT dosimetry in children: the challenge to the pediatric imager. Semin Nucl Med 2007;37:391.

FDG PET Imaging of Large-Vessel Vasculitis

Qi Cao, MD, PhD, Wengan Chen, MD, PhD*

KEYWORDS

- Vasculitis • Giant cell arteritis • Takayasu arteritis
- Polymyalgia rheumatica • [18F]deoxyglucose
- Positron emission tomography

Positron emission tomography (PET) with [18F]deoxyglucose (FDG) is primarily used in cancer staging, restaging, and treatment response evaluation. Data have shown that FDG PET also has a potential role in diagnosing infectious or inflammatory diseases and in monitoring response to therapy. FDG PET may be particularly of value for patients with fever of known origin (FUO).[1] The role of FDG PET for inflammatory vasculitis was initially discovered when FDG PET was compared with gallium scintigraphy for diagnosing FUO a decade ago.

FDG accumulates in activated inflammatory cells due to overexpression of glucose transporters and activation of glycolytic enzymes. In vasculitis there is extensive leukocytic infiltration of the vessel wall, with corresponding reactive damage to regional tissues, which form the biologic basis for FDG PET diagnosis of vasculitis. FDG PET can provide information regarding the extent of the disease or functional impairment, and it is sensitive enough to detect vasculitis in its early stage, well before structural changes become detectable by conventional imaging techniques. This early detection is critical for appropriate clinical management. Although FDG PET has been increasingly used to diagnose vasculitis, its exact clinical significance remains undetermined. This article systemically summarizes recent evidence and achievements regarding the role of FDG PET in the diagnosis and management of vasculitis.

CLINICAL MANIFESTATION, PATHOPHYSIOLOGY, DIAGNOSIS, AND TREATMENT OF VASCULITIS

Vasculitis refers to inflammation of vessel walls and is classified based on the vessel size into large-size vessel, medium-size vessel, and small-size vessel vasculitis.[2] **Table 1** lists the main types of vasculitis under this classification. Although histologic findings are similar, vasculitis can be related to different etiologies. Due to the wide spread of vessels in various organs, the clinical manifestation of vasculitis may be diverse, making diagnosis a challenge. In general, the symptoms of vasculitis are nonspecific, such as focal or entire body pain, fever, and fatigue, although some symptoms are specific in patients with certain types of vasculitis (eg, vision changes in giant cell arteritis [GCA]).

The main pathophysiology of large-size vessel vasculitis lies in the dendritic cells that are situated in the adventitial layer of the tunica media of the aorta and its first- and second-degree branches.[3] The cells can extend to the wall of the vessel that supplies the vasa vasorum. These cells are remnants of immune cells and express toll like receptors (TLRs).[4] When activated, these dendritic cells induce migration of CD4 positive T cells to the tunica media of the blood vessel followed by macrophage invasion, leading to an inflammatory cascade. Release of proinflammatory cytokines such as interleukin (IL)-1 and IL-6 or tumor

The authors have nothing to disclose.
Department of Diagnostic Radiology & Nuclear Medicine, University of Maryland School of Medicine, 22 South Greene Street, Baltimore, MD 21201, USA
* Corresponding author.
E-mail address: wchen5@umm.edu

PET Clin 7 (2012) 227–232
doi:10.1016/j.cpet.2012.01.007

Table 1
Classification of vasculitis

Large-vessel Vasculitis	Medium-size Vessel Vasculitis	Small-vessel Vasculitis (All Varieties not Included)
a. Giant-cell arteritis	a. Polyarteritis nodosa	a. Wegener granulomatosis
b. Takayasu arteritis	b. Kawasaki disease	b. Churg–Strauss syndrome
	c. Primary granulomatous central nervous system vasculitis	c. Henoch–Schönlein purpura
		d. Goodpasture syndrome

necrosis factor-alpha (TNFα) from the activated macrophages leads to symptoms like fever, weight loss, and elevation of plasma erythrocyte sedimentation rate (ESR) and C-reactive protein (CRP). Subsequently, the inflammatory cascade damages the vessel wall, leading to aneurysm formation or dissection.

Diagnosis of vasculitis is challenging given its nonspecific clinic manifestations. Although vascular wall biopsy is 1 of the most reliable methods of diagnosis, it is invasive and has high false-negative results given its difficulty to localize the lesion sites. Laboratory tests such as ESR, CRP, and IL-6 are also nonspecific. Imaging techniques like magnetic resonance imaging (MRI) and ultrasound may be helpful in diagnosis of Takayasu arteritis (TA) and GCA, but their application is limited.

Treatment of vasculitis aims to manage systemic symptoms and suppress vascular inflammation to prevent damage to vessel wall and the tissues they supply. Steroids are the mainstay of treatment, with immunosuppressive agents used for resistant patients or those with steroid-related adverse effects. TNFα antibody such as infliximab and TNFα inhibitor of etanercept have been used in both TA and GCA. Surgical or percutaneous revascularization procedures may be required to improve blood flow or prevent rupture of aneurysms. Angioplasty or surgical repair is required for stenosis, claudication, aneurysms, and dissection of large blood vessels.

FDG PET IN THE DIAGNOSIS OF LARGE-SIZE VESSEL VASCULITIS
Giant Cell Arteritis

GCA is the most common form of vasculitis in Western countries. The prevalence is about 20 cases per 100,000 people older than 50 years of age (female-to-male ratio, 2:1) based on autopsy studies.[5] GCA was initially described as temporal arteritis with a segmental panarteritis in intracranial or extracranial vessels. The thoracic aorta and its main branches are often involved in newly

diagnosed GCA patients. At diagnosis, short-term prognosis is driven by ophthalmic complications that require urgent steroid treatment to prevent the development of definitive blindness.[6] Long-term prognosis is determined by the presence of thoracic aortic aneurysms and stenosis.[7] GCA involving extracranial blood vessels, like the aorta and its major branches, can be visualized by FDG PET scan, which can provide information regarding the extent and depth of vessel wall involvement. In addition, FDG PET can be a useful tool for follow-up of the disease stability and progression. However, its role is limited in intracranial vasculitis given the intense brain FDG uptake and the size of the vessel.

A recent retrospective study[8] including 20 patients and 20 controls showed a sensitivity of 65% and specificity of 80%, yielding an overall diagnostic accuracy of 72% for FDG PET in the diagnosis of large vasculitis. The mean maximum standard uptake value (SUVmax) of the subclavian/carotid region of vasculitis patients was 2.77 ± 1.02, compared with 2.09 ± 0.64 in the control group ($P<.05$). With an SUVmax cut-off value of 1.78, receiver operating characteristic curve (ROC) analysis revealed the highest sensitivity of 90% and specificity of 45%. However, the case number in the study was not sufficient enough to establish generally valid cut-off value. A higher sensitivity of 89%[9] and a higher specificity of 98% have been reported by others.[10] It has been noted that FDG PET has a reduced specificity for vessel wall uptake in the abdominal aorta and lower extremities,[10,11] which could be due to atherosclerosis. The performance of FDG PET for vasculitis may be improved in combining detailed clinical information. **Fig. 1** is an example of a patient with GCA that showed intense vascular wall uptake in the bilateral subclavicular arteries, arch and abdominal aorta, as well as its branches.

In a prospective study involving 35 patients with GCA, vascular FDG uptake was noted in 29 patients (83%), especially in the subclavian arteries (74%), but also in the aorta (>50%) and up to the femoral arteries (37%).[12] There was

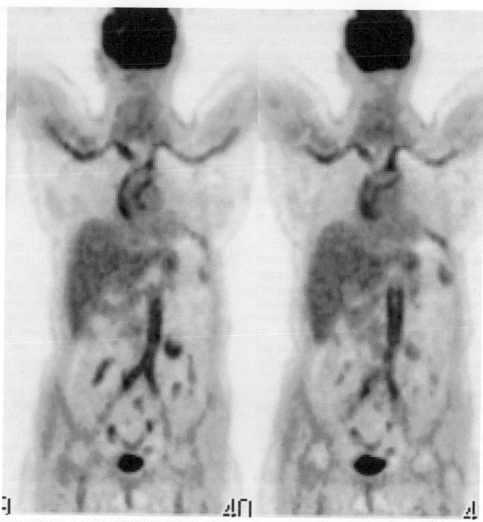

Fig. 1. [18F]deoxyglucose (FDG) positron emission tomography scan obtained from a patient with giant cell arteritis. Extensive vessel wall FDG uptake was noted in the bilateral subclavian arteries, arch, abdominal aorta, and its branches. (*From* Lehmann P, Buchtala S, Achajew N, et al. 18F-FDG PET as a diagnostic procedure in large vessel vasculitis—a controlled, blinded re-examination of routine PET scans. Clin Rheumatol 2011;30:39; with permission.)

significant decrease in vascular FDG uptake on repeat PET scan at 3 months, indicating its potential role in evaluation of treatment response. However, there was no further decrease of vascular wall FDG uptake at 6 months, which could be related to a high metabolic rate during healing, or fibrotic remodeling. There was no correlation of the intensity and extent of FDG uptake at baseline and follow-up to the frequency of relapses, indicating there is no role of a repeating PET scan in identifying patients at risk of relapse.[12] It is worth noting that FDG PET imaging may not be reliable for assessing vasculitis once steroid treatment has been started, as shown in other studies.[13,14]

A prospective study with 46 biopsy-proven GCA patients investigated the potential correlation

between the extent of vascular FDG uptake during the acute phase and the aortic diameter at late follow-up. Patients with increased FDG uptake in the aorta at the diagnosis of GCA had a significantly larger diameter of the ascending aorta, descending aorta, and a significantly larger volume of the thoracic aorta at follow-up. In addition, FDG uptake at the thoracic aorta was the only parameter that was associated with late volume of the thoracic aorta. These findings indicate that FDG PET imaging may play a role in predicting aortic dilatation.[15]

Blockmans and colleagues[14] reported their results of FDG PET scintigraphy in 6 patients with GCA, 5 patients with isolated polymyalgia rheumatic (PMR), and 23 age-matched patients with other inflammatory conditions. Vascular wall FDG uptake was increased in 4 of the 6 GCA patients. Surprisingly, 4 of the 5 PMR patients also showed uptake in their thoracic vessels, indicating the presence of GCA. In contrast, only 1 of 23 controls showed uptake. The results suggest that PET is very helpful to make a diagnosis of GCA in patients with PMR, especially if there are no clinical GCA-related symptoms.

Takayasu Arteritis

TA is a rare disease characterized by chronic and progressive granulomatous inflammatory, fibrotic, and even occlusive vasculitis of the large- and medium-size arteries. In the United States, TA is estimated to affect 2.6 people per million population annually.[16] In Japan and other Asian countries, the incidence is much higher.[16] TA mostly affects young women and presents a diagnostic challenge until advanced stage, when pulseless peripheral arteries become evident. Early stages of the disease show a panarteritis and inflammatory wall thickening of the aorta and its branches, whereas advanced (fibrotic) stages are comprised of stenosis, aneurismatic transformation, and occlusion.

Although angiography is the current gold standard for the diagnosis of advanced stenotic lesions in TA, it is invasive and has a limited role in detecting early stages of the disease. FDG PET imaging is useful as a noninvasive alternative, with great sensitivity in diagnosing early TA.

Meller and colleagues[17] reported successful diagnosis of TA in 5 patients suffering from FUO. FDG PET was subsequently compared with angiography and MRI in 18 patients with suspected TA,[18] which showed that 16 of 18 patients met criteria for TA on FDG PET, leading to a sensitivity of 92%, specificity of 100%, negative predictive value of 85%, and positive predictive value of 100%. FDG PET performance was superior to MRI. In a separate study with 32 TA patients (9 active and 23 inactive disease)[19] compared with disease activity assessed by the National Institutes of Health criteria, PET showed a sensitivity of 78% and a specificity of 87% for active TA. However, low performance of FDG PET for GCA was also reported. Kobayashi and colleagues[20] showed that intense FDG uptake (SUV $\geq$2.7) was noted in only 2 out of 11 active TA patients, with mild uptake in the rest of 9 patients (SUV between 1.2 and 2.3), which made it difficult to identify the location of the disease. Plasma ESR and CRP levels were found to be significantly higher in PET-positive patients than in those with negative PET.[19] In contrast, Arnaud and colleagues[21] reported their experience with 40 PET scans in 28 patients with TA and showed no statistical association between clinical data or levels of acute-phase reactants and intensity of FDG-uptake. The discrepancy may be related to the clinical activity of TA.

Andrews and colleagues[22] followed 6 confirmed cases of TA. After immunosuppressive treatment, 5 patients went into remission, which was associated with a significant decreased FDG uptake in vasculature (**Fig. 2**). In the patient whose TA remained active, FDG uptake remained stable. Kobayashi and colleagues[20] also showed similar findings. Thus, FDG PET may predict the treatment response and disease activity in TA.

FDG PET IN THE DIAGNOSIS OF MEDIUM- AND SMALL-SIZE VESSEL VASCULITIS

Studies regarding the role of FDG PET in the diagnosis of medium- and small-size vessel vasculitis, such as polyarteritis nodosa, lupus erythematosus (SLE), Kawasaki disease, and Wegener granulomatosis, are limited. SLE, polyarteritis nodosa, Kawasaki disease, and Wegener granulomatosis are autoimmune diseases that preferentially affect small- to medium-size arteries. In SLE, cardiac dysfunction was evaluated by FDG PET, in combination with 201thallium chloride for the evaluation of myocardial perfusion.[23] Global perfusion as seen on 201thallium scans was normal in almost all patients, whereas the heart presented an inhomogeneous FDG uptake. Since global perfusion was normal, the authors attributed the focally decreased FDG metabolic process to the presence of a vasculitis process at a level of small capillaries. Central nervous system (CNS) involvement has been found in 30% to 75% of all SLE patients, and clinical diagnosis of CNS lupus has been difficult, given a lack of reliable and sensitive marker for CNS disease activity. FDG PET as a functional imaging technique has been compared with computed tomography (CT) and MRI.

CT and MRI showed only gross abnormalities including edema or small infarcts, both in focal and diffuse CNS lupus. In contrast, FDG PET showed that cerebral blood flow and glucose uptake were decreased during active focal and diffuse CNS lupus.[24] Subsequent studies showed a good correlation between FDG PET and neurologic findings, and PET was considered the most sensitive method for CNS involvement in SLE.[25,26] Applications of FDG PET for CNS involvement in patients with Wegener granulomatosis and polyarteritis nodosa have been reported, but there have been limited case reports.[27]

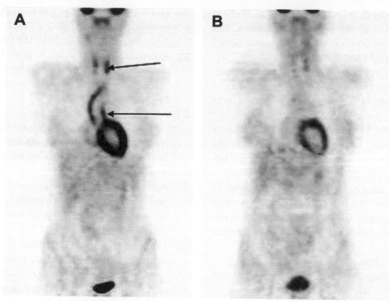

Fig. 2. (A) [18F]deoxyglucose (FDG) positron emission tomography (PET) scan of a patient with active Takayasu arteritis at diagnosis. Note the markedly abnormal uptake of FDG in the aortic arch and carotid arteries (arrows). (B) FDG PET scan of the same patient in remission after treatment with prednisone and intravenous cyclophosphamide. Note almost complete resolution of abnormal [18F]FDG uptake in these areas. (From Andrews J, Al-Nahhas A, Pennell DJ, et al. Non-invasive imaging in the diagnosis and management of Takayasu's arteritis. Ann Rheum Dis 2004;63:998; with permission.)

SUMMARY

Diagnosis of vasculitis is challenging clinically, given its nonspecific symptoms and signs. Although FDG PET has not been included in any vasculitis classification criteria and has not been recommended as a routine diagnostic tool in patients with suspected vasculitis, it is increasingly used in clinic to facilitate the diagnosis of large-vessel vasculitis such as GCA and TA. Accumulating data in the literature support the potential role of FDG PET in the diagnosis of large-vessel vasculitis, in monitoring disease progression, and in assessing treatment response. FDG PET may predict future vessel dilatation caused by vasculitis. However, there appears no definite role of follow-up FDG PET scan in identifying patients at risk of relapse. Application of FDG PET is limited for evaluation of intracranial temporal arteritis, and for medium- as well as small-size vessel vasculitis. It is critical that interpretation of vascular FDG PET uptake should include the clinical context and that the diagnosis of vasculitis should not solely be based on PET.

REFERENCES

1. Meller J, Sahlmann CO, Gurocak O, et al. FDG-PET in patients with fever of unknown origin: the importance of diagnosing large vessel vasculitis. Q J Nucl Med Mol Imaging 2009;53:51–63.

2. Jenette JC, Falk RJ, Andrassy K, et al. Nonmenclature of systemic vasculitides. Proposal of an international consensus conferences. Arthritis Rheum 1994;37:187–92.

3. Han JW, Shimada K, Ma-Krupa W, et al. Vessel wall embedded dendritic cells induce T-cell autoreactivity and initiate vascular inflammation. Circ Res 2008; 102:546–53.

4. Pryshchep O, Ma-Krupa W, Younge BR, et al. Vessel specific Toll-like receptor profile in human medium and large arteries. Circulation 2008;108:1276–84.

5. Ostberg G. An arteritis with special reference to polymyalgia arteritica. Acta Pathol Microbiol Scand Suppl 1973;237:1–59.

6. González-Gay MA, García-Porrúa C, Llorca J, et al. Visual manifestations of giant cell arteritis. Trends and clinical spectrum in 161 patients. Medicine (Baltimore) 2000;79:283–92.

7. Nuenninghoff DM, Hunder GG, Christianson TJ, et al. Incidence and predictors of large-artery complication (aortic aneurysm, aortic dissection, and/or large-artery stenosis) in patients with giant cell arteritis: a population-based study over 50 years. Arthritis Rheum 2003;48:3522–31.

8. Lehmann P, Buchtala S, Achajew N, et al. 18F-FDG PET as a diagnostic procedure in large vessel vasculitis—a controlled, blinded re-examination of routine PET scans. Clin Rheumatol 2011;30:37–42.

9. Hautzel H, Sander O, Heinzel A, et al. Assessment of large-vessel involvement in giant cell arteritis with 18F-FDG PET: introducing an ROC-analysis-based cutoff ratio. J Nucl Med 2008;49:1107–13.

10. Blockmans D, Stroobants S, Maes A, et al. Positron emission tomography in giant cell arteritis and polymyalgia rheumatica: evidence for inflammation of the aortic arch. Am J Med 2000;108:246–9.

11. de Leeuw K, Bijl M, Jager PL. Additional value of positron emission tomography in diagnosis and follow-up of patients with large vessel vasculitides. Clin Exp Rheumatol 2004;22:S21–6.

12. Blockmans D, de Ceuninck L, Vanderschueren S, et al. Repetitive 18F-fluorodeoxyglucose positron emission tomography in giant cell arteritis: a prospective study of 35 patients. Arthritis Rheum 2006;55: 131–7.

13. Blockmans D, Bley T, Schmidt W. Imaging for large-vessel vasculitis. Curr Opin Rheumatol 2009; 21:19–28.

14. Blockmans D, Maes A, Stroobants S, et al. New arguments for a vasculitic nature of polymyalgia rheumatica using positron emission tomography. Rheumatology 1999;38:444–51.

15. Blockmans D, Coudyzer W, Vanderschueren S, et al. Relationship between fluorodeoxyglucose uptake in the large vessels and late aortic diameter in giant cell arteritis. Rheumatology 2008;47:1179–84.

16. Richards BL, March L, Gabriel SE. Epidemiology of large-vessel vasculidities. Best Pract Res Clin Rheumatol 2010;24:871–83.

17. Meller J, Grabbe E, Becker W, et al. Value of F-18 FDG hybrid camera PET and MRI in early Takayasu aortitis. Eur Radiol 2003;13:400–5.

18. Webb M, Chambers A, AL-Nahhas A, et al. The role of 18F-FDG PET in characterising disease activity in Takayasu arteritis. Eur J Nucl Med Mol Imaging 2004;31:627–34.

19. Lee SG, Ryu JS, Kim HO, et al. Evaluation of disease activity using F-18 FDG PET-CT in patients with Takayasu arteritis. Clin Nucl Med 2009;34:749–52.

20. Kobayashi Y, Ishii K, Oda K, et al. Aortic wall inflammation due to Takayasu arteritis imaged with 18F-FDG PET coregistered with enhanced CT. J Nucl Med 2005;46:917–22.

21. Arnaud L, Haroche J, Malek Z, et al. Is 18Ffluorodeoxyglucose positron emission tomography scanning a reliable way to assess disease activity in Takayasu arteritis? Arthritis Rheum 2009;60: 1193–200.

22. Andrews J, Al-Nahhas A, Pennell DJ, et al. Non-invasive imaging in the diagnosis and management of Takayasu's arteritis. Ann Rheum Dis 2004;63: 995–1000.

23. Moncayo R, Kowald E, Schauer N, et al. Detection of myocardial involvement in systemic lupus erythematosus: mismatch between normal perfusion scans with 201thallium and pathological 18FDG uptake. Int Angiol 2001;20:314–21.

24. Kao CH, Ho YJ, Lan JL, et al. Discrepancy between regional cerebral blood flow and glucose metabolism of the brain in systemic lupus erythematosus patients with normal brain magnetic resonance imaging findings. Arthritis Rheum 1999;42:61–8.

25. Stoppe G, Wildhagen K, Seidel JW, et al. Positron emission tomography in neuropsychiatric lupus erythematosus. Neurology 1990;40:304–8.

26. Weiner SM, Otte A, Schumacher M, et al. Alterations of cerebral glucose metabolism indicate progress to severe morphological brain lesions in neuropsychiatric systemic lupus erythematosus. Lupus 2000;9: 386–9.

27. Marienhagen J, Geissler A, Lang B. High resolution single photon emission computed tomography of the brain in Wegener's granulomatosis. J Rheumatol 1996;23:1828–30.

Assessment of Therapy Response by FDG PET in Infection and Inflammation

Rakesh Kumar, MD, PhD[a,*], Sellam Karunanithi, MD[a], Hongming Zhuang, MD, PhD[b], Abass Alavi, MD, PhD (Hon), DSc (Hon)[c]

KEYWORDS

- [18]F FDG-PET • Vasculitis • Magnetic resonance imaging

Early diagnosis or exclusion of infection/inflammation is of importance for the optimal management of patients with such infection or inflammation. Whole-body imaging with fluorodeoxyglucose F 18 (FDG)-PET for the diagnosis, staging, monitoring of response to treatment, and detecting recurrent malignant diseases has been well established.[1–3] The introduction of PET/computed tomography (CT) has added a major dimension to FDG-PET imaging. Despite great successes achieved by FDG-PET imaging in the evaluation of malignant disorders, the test is not specific for cancer. Benign processes, such as infection, inflammation, and granulomatous diseases, appear to have increased glycolysis and are therefore readily visualized by FDG-PET imaging. High tissue radioactivity after the administration of FDG corresponds to increased glucose uptake and consumption through the hexose monophosphate shunt, the main source of energy in chemotaxis and phagocytosis. Activation of phagocytes, also known as respiratory burst activation, leads to increased uptake of FDG. In sterile inflammation, administered FDG is mainly taken up by neutrophils and macrophages. Overexpression of glucose transporter 1 receptors in stimulated macrophages, neutrophils, and lymphocytes is considered the most likely underlying biological phenomenon responsible for this observation.[4,5] The tracer accumulation depends on the degree of stimulation.

PET is a well-known imaging modality in assessing the treatment response to chemotherapy or radiotherapy in various malignancies.[6,7] A systematic review of the literature reveals a few publications reporting the evaluation of treatment response in benign conditions using PET/CT. PET holds a promising future role in the follow-up of inflammatory or infectious diseases. FDG-PET as a tool in the evaluation, treatment, and follow-up of infectious and inflammatory diseases is discussed in this article.

OVERVIEW OF PET IN INFECTION OR INFLAMMATION

A PET scan, being a functional imaging modality, is expected to be useful in early detection, in delineating the actual lesion, and in monitoring the treatment response when compared with conventional imaging, such as CT, magnetic resonance (MR) imaging, and ultrasonography (US). Unlike CT, a PET scan is safe and noninvasive (no contrast used) and, unlike MR imaging, can be used in patients with metallic implants. The role

[a] Department of Nuclear Medicine, All India Institute of Medical Sciences, New Delhi 110029, India
[b] Division of Nuclear Medicine, Department of Radiology, The Children's Hospital of Philadelphia, University of Pennsylvania School of Medicine, 34th Street and Civic Center Boulevard, Philadelphia, PA 19104, USA
[c] Division of Nuclear Medicine, Department of Radiology, Hospital of the University of Pennsylvania, 3400 Spruce Street, Philadelphia, PA 19104, USA
* Corresponding author.
E-mail address: rkphulia@yahoo.com

PET Clin 7 (2012) 233–243
doi:10.1016/j.cpet.2012.01.004

of FDG-PET was demonstrated in 1987, when Theron and Tyler[8] reported the usefulness of FDG-PET in the diagnosis and treatment of Takayasu arteritis (TA). In the next 1.5 decades, many investigators reported the increased uptake of FDG in various infectious or inflammatory lesions. Tissue sites with active infections that excite host inflammatory responses take up larger amounts of FDG than do similar but unaffected surrounding sites. FDG-PET imaging has a major role in the oncologic setting. However, more recently FDG-PET has been gaining wider acceptance in the diagnosis and management of inflammatory processes, which is due to a better understanding of the immunohistopathology underlying the inflammatory mechanism, and the so-called respiratory burst that occurs when resting cells are activated in response to phagocytes (ie, neutrophils, eosinophils, and mononuclear phagocytes) and start metabolizing large quantities of glucose with increased rates of oxygen uptake, sometimes more than 50-fold.[9] Thus, uptake of FDG, a radioactively tagged glucose analogue that cannot be metabolized, is enhanced at such sites because the glycolytic metabolic pathway becomes activated in specialized host cells that mediate inflammatory responses, including polymorphonuclear cells, lymphocytes, and macrophages. Moreover, cytokines stimulate such cells to incorporate higher levels of glucose transporters along the cell surface.

FDG uptake is directly proportional to the level of glycolysis in the cell. Therefore, FDG uptake can be expected to increase in malignant lesions, certain benign lesions, inflammatory lesions, and infectious lesions as well as normally in organs, such as the brain, heart, and endometrium. The uptake is nonspecific, however, and it can sometimes be difficult to differentiate between benign and malignant lesions as well as between infections and sterile inflammation. Inflammatory lesions are known to cause misinterpretation of the findings in patients with malignancy, usually arising as post-biopsy inflammation. Several investigators have suggested dual-time-point PET to differentiate between malignancy and inflammation.[10–12] Malignant lesions typically have increased uptake of FDG for several hours before a peak standard uptake value (SUV) is reached, whereas FDG uptake is reduced in inflammatory lesions over time. The results of various reports on breast, lung, and head and neck cancers support these predictions.[10–12] Kumar and colleagues[11] demonstrated an average increase of 12.6% in SUV between the 2 time points in breast cancer. Conversely, inflammation showed a decrease in the average SUV of −10.2% over time. The

investigators reported a cutoff value of 3.75 or more in SUV in differentiating inflammatory and malignant lesions. Similarly, in head and neck cancers, Hustinx and colleagues[12] reported an average increase of 23% in SUV between the 2 time points. Sites of inflammation had SUV changes that varied from −2.4% to 2.8%, which was significantly less than the SUV changes seen in the malignant lesions. In addition to the early detection of inflammation, the future holds great promise for the role of FDG-PET in the follow-up of patients with inflammatory lesions, whether they are sterile inflammatory lesions or infectious lesions. FDG-PET demonstrates early change as a decreased uptake of FDG if the inflammatory lesions respond to treatment. Conversely, FDG-PET shows persistently increased uptake if the inflammatory lesions do not respond to treatment. The evolution of FDG uptake reflects the efficacy of the medical treatment, and its careful assessment can lead to a better modulation of the drug dosage or prompt a radical modification of the therapeutic strategy.

VASCULITIS

In 1987, Theron and Tyler[8] reported on the usefulness of FDG-PET in the diagnosis and treatment of a case of TA. Since then, many investigators have supported the role of FDG-PET in patients with vasculitis, especially TA and giant-cell arteritis (GCA).[13–26] In addition to early diagnosis, another important aspect in the management of vasculitis is detecting the treatment response as early as possible so that early intervention can be instituted appropriately. Many investigators have reported on the usefulness of FDG-PET in determining whether there is an appropriate response to therapy in the follow-up of patients with vasculitis, and have evaluated the correlation between FDG vascular uptake and serologic levels of inflammatory markers (**Table 1**). A decrease in serologic levels of inflammatory markers and FDG vascular uptake under immunosuppressive treatment has been described during the follow-up for patients with vasculitis, but the disease activity and the risk of relapse do not seem to correlate with the PET findings under therapy.

Meller and colleagues[19] compared FDG-PET/CT with MR imaging, and found FDG-PET/CT to be superior in monitoring disease activity during immunosuppressive therapy in patients with GCA. The anatomic changes associated with vasculitis seen on MR imaging (such as vessel-wall thickening) lag behind improvement in laboratory findings and clinical symptoms. FDG-PET has also been shown to more accurately demonstrate the

Table 1
FDG-PET studies for diagnosis and evaluation of the treatment response in patients with vasculitis

Study No.	References	Type of Study	Patients Evaluated with PET	Diagnosis	Correlation Between PET with Serologic Markers of Inflammation
1	Theron and Tyler,[8] 1987	Case report	1	TA	NR
2	Derdelinckx et al,[17] 2000	Case report	1	Aortitis	NR
3	Turlakow et al,[18] 2001	Case report	1	GCA	NR
4	Meller et al,[19] 2003	Evaluation study	6	GCA	NR
5	Bleeker-Rovers et al,[21] 2003	Evaluation study	5	PAN + GCA + WG	NR
6	de Leeuw et al,[23] 2004	Case series	5	GCA + TA	NR
7	Bleeker-Rovers et al,[22] 2004	Case reports	3	PAN + WG + GCA	NR
8	Webb et al,[24] 2004	Evaluation study	8	TA	NR
9	Andrews et al,[25] 2004	Evaluation study	6	TA	NR
10	Scheel et al,[26] 2004	Evaluation study	8	Aortitis	Correlation
11	Moreno et al,[20] 2005	Case reports	2	TA	NR
12	Blockmans et al,[27] 2006	Evaluation study	35	GCA or PMR	No significant correlation
13	Nakajo et al,[28] 2007	Evaluation study	6	RF	NR
14	Blockmans et al,[29] 2008	Evaluation study	46	GCA	NR
15	Both et al,[30] 2008	Evaluation study	25	GCA	No significant correlation
16	Janssen et al,[31] 2008	Evaluation study	9	GCA	NR
17	Bruschi et al,[32] 2008	Evaluation study	25	NR	No significant correlation
18	Hautzel et al,[33] 2008	Evaluation study	18	GCA	NR
19	Henes et al,[34] 2008	Evaluation study	13	GCA	No significant correlation
20	Arnaud et al,[35] 2009	Evaluation study	28	TA	No significant correlation
21	Lee et al,[36] 2009	Evaluation study	32	TA	Correlation
22	Bertagna et al,[37] 2010	Evaluation study	9	TA	Correlation
23	Piccoli et al,[38] 2010	Evaluation study	7	RF	No significant correlation
24	Jansen et al,[39] 2010	Evaluation study	26	RF	Correlation
25	Lehmann et al,[40] 2011	Evaluation study	20	17 GCA + 3 TA	NR
26	Pfadenhauer et al,[41] 2011	Evaluation study	46	GCA	NR
27	Papathanasiou et al,[42] 2011	Evaluation study	34	NR	Correlation

Abbreviations: GCA, giant-cell arteritis; NR, not reported; PAN, polyarteritis nodosa; PMR, polymyalgia rheumatica; RF, retroperitoneal fibrosis; TA, Takayasu arteritis; WG, Wegener granulomatosis.

extent of disease and monitor disease activity during immunosuppressive therapy (**Fig. 1**). Also during follow-up, FDG uptake showed good correlation with inflammatory markers and clinical symptoms.[19] This finding suggests that FDG-PET/CT can reliably detect the earliest changes of disease improvement after therapy, and persistent activity is an indicator of nonresponders to therapy.[19] In 2006, Blockmans and colleagues[27] evaluated 35 patients with GCA at diagnosis,

during steroid treatment, and at time of relapse. Vascular FDG uptake was reduced at FDG-PET scan performed after 3 months ($P<.0005$) but was not further decreased at 6-month follow-up. The patients in whom GCA relapsed had similar FDG uptake reductions between the baseline and the follow-up PET scan compared with the patients in whom GCA did not relapse. The investigators concluded that increased FDG uptake of the large vessels is a sensitive marker for GCA

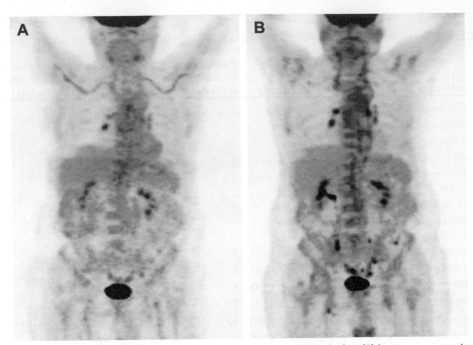

Fig. 1. FDG-PET maximum-intensity projection (MIP) images before (*A*) and after (*B*) immunosuppressive (steroid) therapy in a 73-year-old man with GCA. At baseline (*A*), FDG-PET showed increased FDG uptake in the vessel wall of the subclavian and axillary vessels, consistent with large-vessel vasculitis. The increased vascular FDG uptake disappeared after immunosuppressive therapy (*B*), suggesting a resolution of the inflammatory process.

and that FDG-PET does not predict the relapse of GCA.[27]

The predictive value of clinical and biochemical features compared with FDG-PET in the workup of 25 patients with vasculitis was evaluated by Bruschi and colleagues.[32] Both clinical and biochemical features showed low correlation with FDG-PET findings. A negative correlation between steroid dose and number of scans suggestive for large-vessel vasculitis (LVV) was observed. The investigators found that FDG-PET represents a useful diagnostic tool in the early stages of vasculitis and a powerful instrument to follow the treatment response. Comparison of MR imaging with FDG-PET for the assessment of disease activity in 25 patients with complicated GCA despite immunosuppressive therapy was done by Both and colleagues[30] in 2008. Active disease was detected in 22 and 20 patients by MR imaging and FDG-PET, respectively. Although serologic and clinical findings correlated significantly, there was no concordance with the findings of MR imaging and no significant correlation between FDG-PET and C-reactive protein (CRP) ($P = .136$), erythrocyte sedimentation rate (ESR) ($P = .320$), and clinical findings ($P = .221$). This result suggests that MR imaging and FDG-PET are unreliable for assessing large-vessel inflammation in patients

with complicated GCA during immunosuppressive therapy.[30] Zerizer and colleagues[43] evaluated the role of FDG-PET/CT in the diagnosis and management of vasculitis and found that the modality has proven validity in this setting, with sensitivity values ranging from 77% to 92% and specificities ranging from 89% to 100%. FDG-PET/CT has proven use in the initial diagnosis of patients suspected of having vasculitis, particularly those who present with nonspecific symptoms; in the identification of areas of increased FDG uptake requiring biopsy; and in the evaluation of the extent of disease.

Pfadenhauer and colleagues[41] evaluated the ability of FDG-PET to detect active GCA of the extracerebral vertebral artery (VA) in a comparison with clinical, US, and biopsy findings in 46 patients. FDG-PET was superior to US for the detection of active GCA, including VA involvement, because 15 of the 46 (33%) patients with GCA had abnormal FDG uptake of the VA. In 2 of the 15 patients (4%), increased FDG uptake of a single VA was the only PET abnormality, whereas in 13 of the 15 patients, a concomitant increased FDG uptake of the large arteries was observed. A strong correlation between PET abnormalities in VA and clinical abnormalities was observed in two-thirds of the patients. Abnormal vascular FDG uptake was detectable in 5 patients despite glucocorticoid treatment. The investigators concluded that abnormal FDG uptake of the VA can be an early and isolated finding of active GCA, and can be detected in some cases despite steroid treatment.[41]

The diagnostic performance of FDG-PET/CT in 78 patients with suspected LVV was investigated by Papathanasiou and colleagues.[42] Three clinically classified groups, (1) steroid-naive LVV (16 patients), (2) LVV on steroid treatment (18 patients), and (3) no evidence of LVV (44 patients), were evaluated. FDG-PET/CT result was positive in patients with steroid-naive LVV, and in these patients FDG vascular uptake was significantly higher than in other groups ($P<.05$). A significant positive association ($P<.05$) was found between FDG uptake of the thoracic aorta and inflammatory markers in patients with LVV. The patients on steroid treatment showed lower FDG vascular uptake than steroid-naive patients. These findings demonstrated that FDG-PET/CT can detect the extent and activity of LVV in untreated patients, but that it is unreliable for LVV diagnosis in patients on steroid treatment.[42]

TA is rare, affecting 2 to 3 patients per million population worldwide.[44] It predominantly affects young women (age range 15–20 years) and characteristically presents with a chronic, progressive, inflammatory, occlusive disease of the aorta and its branches, predominantly the subclavian vessels and also the pulmonary arteries in up to 50% of patients.[44] Lee and colleagues[36] evaluated the usefulness of FDG-PET/CT in detecting active disease in 32 patients with TA. Ten patients had active lesions on FDG-PET/CT, showing a high-grade linear FDG uptake along the aortic wall. Compared with the clinical disease-activity criteria, FDG-PET/CT had a sensitivity of 78% and a specificity of 87%. Although the specificity of FDG-PET/CT was high, in interpreting these findings the clinical disease-activity criteria have low sensitivity in detecting pathologically proven active disease.[36] Eight patients with TA detected by FDG-PET/CT before and after corticosteroid treatment were evaluated by Bertagna and colleagues,[37] who demonstrated that this method is an accurate tool for establishing the diagnosis of TA, evaluating disease extension, and monitoring therapy in conjunction with clinical and biochemical findings.[37]

Recently, Jansen and colleagues[39] evaluated whether FDG-PET was useful in the therapeutic evaluation of patients with retroperitoneal fibrosis (RF) treated with tamoxifen. Patients with a positive result on FDG-PET scan had a higher CRP level and a larger mass size at CT scan compared with patients with a negative result on FDG-PET scan. FDG uptake decreased after treatment, in agreement with ESR reduction ($P<.001$), but not

with CT-documented mass regression. These investigators concluded that (1) FDG-PET may be useful to evaluate the severity and the extent of RF, and (2) FDG-PET may be a valuable tool in assessing disease activity during or after treatment in patients with normal inflammatory marker levels and stable residual mass on repeated CT scans.[39]

The limits of FDG-PET/CT need to be taken into account during the interpretation of each study. False-positive results mainly occur because of the observed increased FDG uptake in atherosclerotic vessels. A large prospective study measured the mean SUV in multiple vascular beds in 149 patients without evidence of vasculitis, and the investigators demonstrated that in those older than 60 years the mean SUV can be up to 2.01 ± 0.50.[45] In the follow-up of patients with vasculitis, increased uptake may persist, and it can be difficult to distinguish between subclinical atherosclerosis, persistent disease activity, and post-treatment vascular changes. This is problematic because increased vascular FDG uptake persists several years after the acute phase of the disease, despite treatment with steroids.[46] In small and medium-sized vessel vasculitis, the limited spatial resolution of PET (4–6 mm) does not accurately display the involvement of small and medium-sized vessels. The masking effect of steroid therapy on the FDG vascular uptake should be considered, because an inverse relationship between the dosage of immunosuppressive therapy and the number of FDG-PET scans with positive results has been reported.[32] This relationship has also been observed in a prospective study of 35 patients with GCA in whom there was an initial reduction in FDG uptake 3 months after treatment with steroids.[23] There was persistent activity observed on subsequent follow-up scan at 6 and 12 months. The investigators explained that this persistent uptake may be due to an immune-resistant response in the arterial wall to steroid therapy, or because of tissue repair and remodeling.[23] FDG-PET and PET/CT findings should be integrated with clinical, serologic, and radiologic findings to achieve the correct management of patients with LVV, because use of SUV alone to diagnose vasculitis can result in a high rate of false-positive results.[47]

BONE INFECTIONS

Bone infections can be acute or chronic. Diagnosis is usually made on clinical grounds and is aided by biochemical parameters, plain radiographs, bone scintigraphy, and MR imaging. FDG-PET/CT, used in combination with conventional methods, may have limited value in the diagnosis of uncomplicated cases of acute osteomyelitis; but may play an important role in patients with chronic osteomyelitis, particularly those with previously documented osteomyelitis and suspected recurrence or presenting with symptoms of osteomyelitis for more than 6 weeks. Kalicke and colleagues[48] evaluated the role of FDG-PET in acute and chronic osteomyelitis and inflammatory spondylitis, and found that FDG-PET was clearly superior to bone scintigraphy for the diagnosis of bone infection. Koort and colleagues[49] conducted an experimental study to evaluate whether FDG-PET can differentiate between a normal bone healing and the healing of a bone with local osteomyelitis. The investigators concluded that FDG-PET was clearly beneficial in differentiating between infection and sterile inflammation or sterile stress fractures in patients with metallic implants and prostheses. A meta-analysis study showed that FDG-PET is not only the most sensitive imaging modality for detecting chronic osteomyelitis, but also has a greater specificity than radiolabeled white blood cell (WBC) scintigraphy, bone scintigraphy, or MR imaging.[50]

In a retrospective study, FDG-PET/CT had a major impact on the clinical management (initiation or prolongation of antibiotic therapy or recourse to surgical intervention) of 52% of patients with infectious spondylitis.[51] A recent review highlights the clinical role of FDG-PET/CT in diagnosing spinal infections, especially in patients with contraindications to MR imaging, and in the evaluation of the postoperative spine.[52] Thus the use of FDG-PET/CT is clearly indicated in spondylodiscitis, even though there is a need for clearer criteria for positivity and for clarification of the role of the standard uptake volume.

In diabetic foot infection, FDG-PET/CT was found to be highly sensitive in excluding osteomyelitis in the diabetic foot, and to usefully complement MR imaging, particularly in cases with positive findings on MR imaging. Conventional imaging, such as MR imaging or bone scanning, lacks specificity in distinguishing osteomyelitis in the diabetic foot from Charcot neuroarthropathy. In a recent prospective study conducted in 110 patients with complicated diabetic foot, FDG-PET/CT was found to be a highly specific imaging modality for the diagnosis of osteomyelitis, and was deemed a useful complementary imaging modality for use with MR imaging.[53]

PROSTHESIS INFECTION

Superimposed infection in prosthetic implants needs to be detected at the earliest possible opportunity so that appropriate intervention can be instituted. A significant long term complication

of hip arthroplasty is aseptic loosening, which can even lead to prosthesis reimplantation. Aseptic loosening and superimposed infections are sometimes difficult to differentiate. Various nuclear medicine techniques, such as leukocyte scans, sulfur colloid bone marrow scans, bone scintigraphy, and FDG-PET scans, have been used in attempts to differentiate between these 2 conditions.[54–56] An earlier study[57] investigated 2 groups of patients with arthroplasty to assess the patterns and time course of FDG accumulation after total hip replacement over an extended period. The investigators concluded that after hip arthroplasty, nonspecific increased FDG uptake around the head or neck of the prosthesis persists for many years, even in patients without any complications. FDG uptake is also increased in sterile inflammation secondary to surgery. FDG-PET is not affected by artifacts caused by metal implants, and provides images with higher resolution than those produced using conventional nuclear medicine techniques. However, noninfectious reactions around the neck of the prosthesis are common months and even years after surgery, and these may influence the diagnosis. Increased FDG uptake around the neck and/or head should not be interpreted as a finding suggestive of infection. Although 10% of patients with hip arthroplasty suffer from significant pain, only 1% is found to have periprosthetic infection after initial surgery, whereas the remainder has prosthetic loosening without infection. The differentiation of mechanical loosening from superimposed infection is a challenge. Chacko and colleagues[58] found that quantification of FDG uptake is not always a good parameter for the evaluation of FDG-PET when characterizing infections. These investigators studied the location and intensity of FDG uptake in 41 total hip arthroplasties from 32 patients, with a complete clinical follow-up. By contrast, images from sterile loose hip prostheses revealed intense uptake around the head or neck of the prosthesis, with SUVs as high as 7. The study concluded that the intensity of increased FDG uptake is less important than the location of the increased FDG uptake when FDG-PET is used to diagnose periprosthetic infection in patients with hip arthroplasty. Studies in the past that compared WBC imaging with FDG-PET scanning in prosthetic joint infections showed better results with WBC imaging, which proved more sensitive and more specific than FDG-PET. The lack of specificity of the FDG-PET/CT modality prompted definition of interpretation criteria.[59] As of now the potential for FDG-PET in the evaluation of prostheses is well defined. More research may further enhance the role of FDG-PET in the evaluation of prostheses. At present, the site and patterns of FDG accumulation seem to be more important than the intensity of uptake at these locations. A recent meta-analysis indicated that the FDG-PET sensitivity in identifying hip prosthesis infections was 82.8%, with specificity of 87.3%. PET based on FDG could be a valid option if research is able to find an uptake pattern specific for septic and aseptic loosening.[60]

OTHER INFECTIONS

Kotilainen and colleagues[61] reported the case of a 41-year-old patient with Riedel thyroiditis, in whom FDG-PET demonstrated intensive FDG uptake in both lobes of the thyroid gland as an indication of severe inflammation. On follow-up of corticosteroid treatment after 2 weeks, an FDG-PET scan showed a 60% decrease in the uptake of FDG in the thyroid. Tsuyuguchi and colleagues[62] evaluated FDG-PET and ^{11}C-methionine PET before and after treatment in 4 patients with a brain abscess. After treatment, the lesion area became small on enhancement with CT or MR imaging, and PET studies showed a reduced lesion size with decreased radiotracer uptake. The investigators concluded that PET was useful in detecting the inflammatory lesion and assessing the clinical effects of antibiotic treatment on brain abscesses. Bleeker-Rovers and colleagues[63] studied FDG-PET scans in 3 patients with adult polycystic kidney diseases with the suspicion of renal or hepatic cyst infection, and the follow-up FDG-PET scan was normal after 6 weeks of successful antibiotic treatment for hepatic cyst infection. Win and colleagues[64] reported a case of *Pneumocystis carinii* pneumonia in a 26-year-old man with moderate to severe leukopenia. FDG-PET demonstrated acute lung changes, which disappeared on the follow-up scan after treatment. The investigators proposed that FDG-PET might prove useful in the diagnosis and evaluation of the treatment response in patients with *P carinii* pneumonia. Ozsahin and colleagues[65] showed that after successful therapy for invasive aspergillosis, FDG-PET findings reverted to normal. In a clinical study, FDG uptake returned to normal levels after successful antibiotic therapy for hepatic cyst infection[63] and after antifungal therapy for a lung abscess caused by candidal infection.[66] FDG-PET has also been reported to be reliable in assessing metabolic activity and in detecting relapses of infection in patients with alveolar echinococcosis.[67]

Because bone scintigraphy detects reactive osteoblastic activity after the initiation of the disease process to the adjacent marrow or other tissues and FDG-PET detects the disease process directly, the time intervals for images acquired by

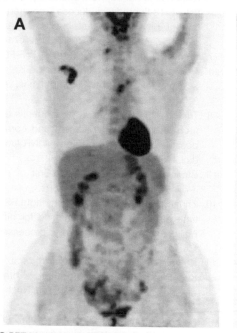
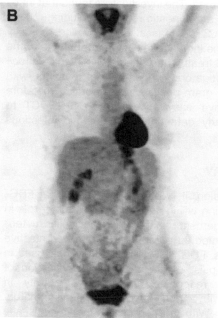

Fig. 2. FDG-PET MIP images before (*A*) and after (*B*) antituberculosis treatment (ATT) in a 51-year-old woman with tuberculosis. Baseline study (*A*) shows intense FDG uptake in mediastinal, right axillary, and right supraclavicular lymph nodes. Follow-up study after 8 weeks of ATT (*B*) shows complete resolution in previously involved sites, suggesting significant response to ATT.

these 2 modalities to return to normal after successful treatment of osteomyelitis vary considerably. An interesting investigation by Hakim and colleagues[68] compared the specificities of these 2 modalities in the evaluation of chronic osteomyelitis of the mandible after the treatment of 42 patients. The specificity of bone scintigraphy was only 6.6%, compared with a specificity of 80% for FDG-PET,[68] which suggests that during the follow-up period bone scintigraphy should be replaced by FDG-PET.[68] FDG-PET holds great promise in the evaluation of treatment response, akin to what it has demonstrated in the evaluation of treatment response in several malignancies. A decrease of 50% in the baseline FDG uptake after antibiotic treatment is considered to be a significant response. Mycobacterial infection can result in elevated FDG activity[69,70] and cause difficulty in interpretation when PET is used to evaluate patients with cancer. However, the change in FDG activity after antibiotic treatment is an effective way of knowing the efficacy of the antituberculosis therapy.[71–73] The response to antituberculosis treatment can be well monitored by FDG-PET/CT (**Fig. 2**).

COST-EFFECTIVENESS OF FDG-PET/CT

Recently, a cost-effectiveness analysis by Vos and colleagues,[74] in a prospective FDG-PET/CT group (n = 115) and matched control group (n = 230), was performed. The investigators found that introduction of a diagnostic regimen including routine FDG-PET/CT decreases morbidity and mortality and that the increase in cost is attributable to the in-hospital treatment of metastatic infectious foci. The investigators proposed that patients with high-risk gram-positive bacteremia therefore should have easy access to FDG-PET/CT to enable early detection of metastatic infectious disease.

SUMMARY

In conclusion, it is becoming evident that FDG-PET imaging will increasingly play a major role in the management of patients with vasculitis, osteomyelitis, infected prostheses, and other infective conditions. FDG-PET will be increasingly used in the diagnosis, extent of disease, evaluation of treatment response, and disease activity in patients with various infectious and inflammatory diseases. With the ability to monitor disease activity and quantify the degree of abnormal metabolism, PET might prove to be an appropriate modality for assessing response to therapy. FDG-PET imaging has shown promising results and

should be used in the clinical management of infectious disorders for optimal outcome of the affected patients, which will substantially improve the management of patients with serious infectious disorders.

REFERENCES

1. Kumar R, Nadig MR, Chauhan A. Positron emission tomography: clinical applications in oncology. Part 1. Expert Rev Anticancer Ther 2005;5:1079–94.
2. Kostakoglu L, Agress H Jr, Goldsmith SJ. Clinical role of FDG PET in evaluation of cancer patients. Radiographics 2003;23:315–40.
3. Kumar R, Bhargava P, Bozkurt MF, et al. Positron emission tomography imaging in evaluation of cancer patients. Indian J Cancer 2003;40:87–100.
4. Fu Y, Maianu L, Melbert BR, et al. Facilitative glucose transporter gene expression in human lymphocytes, monocytes, and macrophages: a role for GLUT isoforms 1, 3, and 5 in the immune response and foam cell formation. Blood Cells Mol Dis 2004;32:182–90.
5. Zhao S, Kuge Y, Tsukamoto E, et al. Fluorodeoxyglucose uptake and glucose transporter expression in experimental inflammatory lesions and malignant tumours: effects of insulin and glucose loading. Nucl Med Commun 2002;23:545–50.
6. Avril N, Sassen S, Schmalfeldt B, et al. Prediction of response to neoadjuvant chemotherapy by sequential F-18-fluorodeoxyglucose positron emission tomography in patients with advanced-stage ovarian cancer. J Clin Oncol 2005;23:7445–53.
7. Kumar R, Xiu Y, Potenta S, et al. ^{18}F-FDG PET for evaluation of the treatment response in patients with gastrointestinal tract lymphomas. J Nucl Med 2004;45:1796–803.
8. Theron J, Tyler JL. Takayasu's arteritis of the aortic arch: endovascular treatment and correlation with positron emission tomography. AJNR Am J Neuroradiol 1987;8:621–6.
9. Babior BM. The respiratory burst of phagocytes. J Clin Invest 1984;73(3):599–601.
10. Zhuang H, Pourdehnad M, Lambright ES, et al. Dual time point ^{18}F-FDG PET imaging for differentiating malignant from inflammatory processes. J Nucl Med 2001;42:1412–7.
11. Kumar R, Loving VA, Chauhan A, et al. Potential of dual-time-point imaging to improve breast cancer diagnosis with (18)F-FDG PET. J Nucl Med 2005; 46:1819–24.
12. Hustinx R, Smith RJ, Benard F, et al. Dual time point fluorine-18 fluorodeoxyglucose positron emission tomography: a potential method to differentiate malignancy from inflammation and normal tissue in the head and neck. Eur J Nucl Med 1999;26:1345–8.

13. Hara M, Goodman PC, Leder RA. FDG-PET finding in early-phase Takayasu arteritis. J Comput Assist Tomogr 1999;23:16–8.

14. Meller J, Grabbe E, Becker W, et al. Value of F-18 FDG hybrid camera PET and MRI in early Takayasu aortitis. Eur Radiol 2003;13:400–5.

15. Brodmann M, Lipp RW, Passath A, et al. The role of 2-F-18-fluoro-2-deoxy-D-glucose positron emission tomography in the diagnosis of giant cell arteritis of the temporal arteries. Rheumatology (Oxford) 2004;43:241–2.

16. Balan K, Voutnis D, Groves A. Discordant uptake of F-18 FDG and In-111 WBC in systemic vasculitis. Clin Nucl Med 2003;28:485–6.

17. Derdelinckx I, Maes A, Bogaert J, et al. Positron emission tomography scan in the diagnosis and follow-up of aortitis of the thoracic aorta. Acta Cardiol 2000;55:193–5.

18. Turlakow A, Yeung HW, Pui J, et al. Fludeoxyglucose positron emission tomography in the diagnosis of giant cell arteritis. Arch Intern Med 2001;161:1003–7.

19. Meller J, Strutz F, Siefker U, et al. Early diagnosis and follow-up of aortitis with [(18)F]FDG PET and MRI. Eur J Nucl Med Mol Imaging 2003;30:730–6.

20. Moreno D, Yuste JR, Rodriguez M, et al. Positron emission tomography use in the diagnosis and follow up of Takayasu's arteritis. Ann Rheum Dis 2005;64:1091–3.

21. Bleeker-Rovers CP, Bredie SJ, van der Meer JW, et al. F-18-fluorodeoxyglucose positron emission tomography in diagnosis and follow-up of patients with different types of vasculitis. Neth J Med 2003;61:323–9.

22. Bleeker-Rovers CP, Bredie SJ, van der Meer JW, et al. Fluorine 18 fluorodeoxyglucose positron emission tomography in the diagnosis and follow-up of three patients with vasculitis. Am J Med 2004;116:50–3.

23. de Leeuw K, Bijl M, Jager PL. Additional value of positron emission tomography in diagnosis and follow-up of patients with large vessel vasculitides. Clin Exp Rheumatol 2004;22(Suppl):S21–6.

24. Webb M, Chambers A, Al-Nahhas A, et al. The role of ^{18}F-FDG PET in characterising disease activity in Takayasu arteritis. Eur J Nucl Med Mol Imaging 2004;31:627–34.

25. Andrews J, Al-Nahhas A, Pennell DJ, et al. Non-invasive imaging in the diagnosis and management of Takayasu's arteritis. Ann Rheum Dis 2004;63:995–1000.

26. Scheel AK, Meller J, Vosshenrich R, et al. Diagnosis and follow up of aortitis in the elderly. Ann Rheum Dis 2004;63:1507–10.

27. Blockmans D, de Ceuninck L, Vanderschueren S, et al. Repetitive ^{18}F-fluorodeoxyglucose positron emission tomography in giant cell arteritis: a prospective study in 35 patients. Arthritis Rheum 2006;55:131–7.

28. Nakajo M, Jinnouchi S, Tanabe H, et al. ^{18}F-fluorodeoxy glucose positron emission tomography features of

29. Blockmans D, Coudyzer W, Vanderschueren S, et al. Relationship between fluorodeoxyglucose uptake in the large vessels and late aortic diameter in giant cell arteritis. Rheumatology 2008;47:1179–84.

30. Both M, Ahmadi-Simab K, Reuter M, et al. MRI and FDG-PET in the assessment of inflammatory aortic arch syndrome in complicated courses of giant cell arteritis. Ann Rheum Dis 2008;67:1030–3.

31. Janssen SP, Comans EH, Voskuyl AE, et al. Giant cell arteritis: heterogeneity in clinical presentation and imaging results. J Vasc Surg 2008;48:1025–31.

32. Bruschi M, De Leonardis F, Govoni M, et al. [18]F FDG-PET and large vessel vasculitis: preliminary data on 25 patients. Reumatismo 2008;60:212–6.

33. Hautzel H, Sander O, Heinzel A, et al. Assessment of large-vessel involvement in giant cell arteritis with ^{18}F-FDG PET: introducing an ROC-analysis-based cutoff ratio. J Nucl Med 2008;49:1107–13.

34. Henes JC, Müller M, Krieger J, et al. [^{18}F] FDG-PET/CT as a new and sensitive imaging method for the diagnosis of large vessel vasculitis. Clin Exp Rheumatol 2008;26(3 Suppl 49):S47–52.

35. Arnaud L, Haroche J, Malek Z, et al. Is (18)F-fluorodeoxyglucose positron emission tomography scanning a reliable way to assess disease activity in Takayasu arteritis? Arthritis Rheum 2009;60:1193–200.

36. Lee SG, Ryu JS, Kim HO, et al. Evaluation of disease activity using F-18 FDG PET CT in patients with Takayasu arteritis. Clin Nucl Med 2009;34:749–52.

37. Bertagna F, Bosio G, Caobelli F, et al. Role of ^{18}F-fluorodeoxyglucose positron emission tomography/computed tomography for therapy evaluation of patients with large-vessel vasculitis. Jpn J Radiol 2010;28:199–204.

38. Piccoli GB, Consiglio V, Arena V, et al. Positron emission tomography as a tool for the 'tailored' management of retroperitoneal fibrosis: a nephrourological experience. Nephrol Dial Transplant 2010;25:2603–10.

39. Jansen I, Hendriksz TR, Han SH, et al. (18)F-fluorodeoxyglucose position emission tomography (FDG-PET) for monitoring disease activity and treatment response in idiopathic retroperitoneal fibrosis. Eur J Intern Med 2010;21:216–21.

40. Lehmann P, Buchtala S, Achajew N, et al. ^{18}F-FDG PET as a diagnostic procedure in large vessel vasculitis—a controlled, blinded re-examination of routine PET scans. Clin Rheumatol 2011;30:37–42.

41. Pfadenhauer K, Weinerth J, Hrdina C. Vertebral arteries: a target for FDG-PET imaging in giant cell arteritis? Clinical, ultrasonographic and PET study in 46 patients. Nuklearmedizin 2011;50:28–32.

42. Papathanasiou ND, Du Y, Menezes LJ, et al. ^{18}F-Fluorodeoxyglucose PET/CT in the evaluation of large-vessel vasculitis: diagnostic performance and

idiopathic retroperitoneal fibrosis. J Comput Assist Tomogr 2007;31:539–43.

correlation with clinical and laboratory parameters. Br J Radiol 2011. [Epub ahead of print].

43. Zerizer I, Tan K, Khan S, et al. Role of FDG-PET and PET/CT in the diagnosis and management of vasculitis. Eur J Radiol 2010;73(3):504–9.

44. Watts R, Al-Taiar A, Mooney J, et al. The epidemiology of Takayasu arteritis in the UK. Rheumatology (Oxford) 2009;48(8):1008–11.

45. Bural GG, Torigian DA, Chamroonrat W, et al. FDG-PET is an effective imaging modality to detect and quantify age-related atherosclerosis in large arteries. Eur J Nucl Med Mol Imaging 2008;35(3):562–9.

46. Blockmans D, Bley T, Schmidt W. Imaging for large-vessel vasculitis. Curr Opin Rheumatol 2009;21(1): 19–28.

47. Mueller M, Henes J, Pfannenber C, et al. Diagnosis of vasculitis with F-18 FDG-PET/CT: quantification of arterial wall activity in vasculitis patients and controls [abstract]. J Nucl Med 2007;48(Suppl 2):224.

48. Kalicke T, Schmitz A, Risse JH, et al. Fluorine-18 fluorodeoxyglucose PET in infectious bone diseases: results of histologically confirmed cases. Eur J Nucl Med 2000;27:524–8.

49. Koort JK, Makinen TJ, Knuuti J, et al. Comparative 18F-FDG PET of experimental Staphylococcus aureus osteomyelitis and normal bone healing. J Nucl Med 2004;45:1406–11.

50. Termaat MF, Raijmakers PG, Scholten HJ, et al. The accuracy of diagnostic imaging for the assessment of chronic osteomyelitis: a systematic review and meta-analysis. J Bone Joint Surg Am 2005;87:2464–71.

51. Ito K, Kubota K, Morooka M, et al. Clinical impact of 18F-FDG PET/CT on the management and diagnosis of infectious spondylitis. Nucl Med Commun 2010; 31(8):691–8.

52. Gemmel F, Rijk PC, Collins JM, et al. Expanding role of 18F-fluoro D-deoxyglucose PET and PET/CT in spinal infections. Eur Spine J 2010;19(4):540–51.

53. Nawaz A, Torigian DA, Siegelman ES, et al. Diagnostic performance of FDG-PET, MRI, and plain film radiography (PFR) for the diagnosis of osteomyelitis in the diabetic foot. Mol Imaging Biol 2010; 12(3):335–42.

54. El Espera I, Blondet C, Moullart V, et al. The usefulness of 99mTc sulfur colloid bone marrow scintigraphy combined with 111In leucocyte scintigraphy in prosthetic joint infection. Nucl Med Commun 2004;25:171–5.

55. Joseph TN, Mujtaba M, Chen AL, et al. Efficacy of combined technetium-99m sulfur colloid/indium-111 leukocyte scans to detect infected total hip and knee arthroplasties. J Arthroplasty 2001;16:753–8.

56. Love C, Marwin SE, Tomas MB, et al. Diagnosing infection in the failed joint replacement: a comparison of coincidence detection 18F-FDG and 111In-labeled leukocyte/99mTc-sulfur colloid marrow imaging. J Nucl Med 2004;45:1864–71.

57. Zhuang H, Chacko TK, Hickeson M, et al. Persistent non-specific FDG uptake on PET imaging following hip arthroplasty. Eur J Nucl Med Mol Imaging 2002;29:1328–33.

58. Chacko TK, Zhuang H, Stevenson K, et al. The importance of the location of fluorodeoxyglucose uptake in periprosthetic infection in painful hip prostheses. Nucl Med Commun 2002;23:851–5.

59. Van der Bruggen W, Bleeker-Rovers CP, Boerman OC, et al. PET and SPECT in osteomyelitis and prosthetic bone and joint infections: a systematic review. Semin Nucl Med 2010;40(1):3–15.

60. Zoccali C, Teori G, Salducca N. The role of FDG-PET in distinguishing between septic and aseptic loosening in hip prosthesis: a review of literature. Int Orthop 2009;33:1–5.

61. Kotilainen P, Airas L, Kojo T, et al. Positron emission tomography as an aid in the diagnosis and follow-up of Riedel's thyroiditis. Eur J Intern Med 2004;15: 186–9.

62. Tsuyuguchi N, Sunada I, Ohata K, et al. Evaluation of treatment effects in brain abscess with positron emission tomography: comparison of fluorine-18-fluorodeoxyglucose and carbon-11-methionine. Ann Nucl Med 2003;17:47–51.

63. Bleeker-Rovers CP, de Sevaux RG, van Hamersvelt HW, et al. Diagnosis of renal and hepatic cyst infections by 18-F-fluorodeoxyglucose positron emission tomography in autosomal dominant polycystic kidney disease. Am J Kidney Dis 2003;41:E18–21.

64. Win Z, Todd J, Al-Nahhas A. FDG-PET imaging in Pneumocystis carinii pneumonia. Clin Nucl Med 2005;30:690–1.

65. Ozsahin H, von Planta M, Muller I, et al. Successful treatment of invasive aspergillosis in chronic granulomatous disease by bone marrow transplantation, granulocyte colony-stimulating factor-mobilized granulocytes, and liposomal amphotericin-B. Blood 1998;92:2719–24.

66. Bleeker-Rovers CP, Warris A, Drenth JP, et al. Diagnosis of Candida lung abscesses by 18F-fluorodeoxy glucose positron emission tomography. Clin Microbiol Infect 2005;11:493–5.

67. Reuter S, Buck A, Manfras B, et al. Structured treatment interruption in patients with alveolar echinococcosis. Hepatology 2004;39:509–17.

68. Hakim SG, Bruecker CW, Jacobsen H, et al. The value of FDG-PET and bone scintigraphy with SPECT in the primary diagnosis and follow-up of patients with chronic osteomyelitis of the mandible. Int J Oral Maxillofac Surg 2006;35:809–16.

69. Li YJ, Cai L, Sun HR, et al. Increased FDG uptake in bilateral adrenal tuberculosis appearing like malignancy. Clin Nucl Med 2008;33:191–2.

70. Lin KH, Wang JH, Peng NJ. Disseminated nontuberculous mycobacterial infection mimic metastases on PET/CT scan. Clin Nucl Med 2008;33:276–7.

71. Takalkar AM, Bruno GL, Reddy M, et al. Intense FDG activity in peritoneal tuberculosis mimics peritoneal carcinomatosis. Clin Nucl Med 2007;32: 244–6.

72. Li YJ, Zhang Y, Gao S, et al. Systemic disseminated tuberculosis mimicking malignancy on F-18 FDG PET-CT. Clin Nucl Med 2008;33:49–51.

73. Park IN, Ryu JS, Shim TS. Evaluation of therapeutic response of tuberculoma using F-18 FDG positron emission tomography. Clin Nucl Med 2008;33:1–3.

74. Vos FJ, Bleeker-Rovers CP, Kullberg BJ, et al. Cost-effectiveness of routine ^{18}F-FDG PET/CT in high-risk patients with gram-positive bacteremia. J Nucl Med 2011;52:1673–8.

Index

Note: Page numbers of article titles are in **boldface** type.

A

Angiography, for Takayasu arteritis, 230
Aorta, giant cell arteritis of, 228–230
Arteritis
 giant cell, 228–230, 235–237
 Takayasu, 230, 234, 237
Arthroplasty, infections associated with, **139–150**, 168–169, **238–239**
Aseptic loosening, in arthroplasty, 139–150, 168–169, 238–239
Atherosclerosis, in diabetic foot, 153–154, 159

B

Biopsy, for fever of unknown origin, 182
Bone, sarcoidosis of, 204
Bone healing, versus osteomyelitis, 164–168
Bone scintigraphy
 for arthroplasty-associated infections, 145
 for diabetic foot, 154, 174
 for osteomyelitis, 163, 166, 171, 237–238, 240
Brain abscess, 239
Brain tumors, inflammation in, 213

C

Cancer
 as source of fever of unknown origin, 185
 infections and inflammation in, **211–218**
Cardiac catheterization, for sarcoidosis, 200
Cardiac sarcoidosis, 200–202
Charcot arthropathy, 152, 158, 173–177, 238
[11C]-Choline, for sarcoidosis, 202
Cierny classification, of osteomyelitis, 164
Colitis, ulcerative, **219–225**
Coronary angiography, for sarcoidosis, 200
Critical illness, fever of unknown origin in, 185
Crohn disease, **219–225**
CT. *See also* PET and PET/CT.
 for diabetic foot, 154
 for fever of unknown origin, 182
 for sarcoidosis, 192
CT enterography, for inflammatory bowel disease, 221–222
CT/SPECT, for osteomyelitis, 163

D

Deep soft tissue infections, in diabetic foot, 152
3'-Deoxy-3'-[18F]-fluorothymidine (FLT), for sarcoidosis, 199
Diabetic foot, PET and PET/CT for, **151–160**, 175
 in atherogenesis evaluation, 173–177
 in Charcot arthropathy, 152, 158
 in deep soft tissue infection, 152
 in ischemia, 153–154
 in osteomyelitis, 152, 154–158, 173–177, 238
 published data on, 156–159
 versus existing techniques, 154–156
Diphosphates, radiolabeled, for osteomyelitis, 163–164
Dosimetry, of radiation, in inflammatory bowel disease, 222, 224

E

Endocarditis, as source of fever of unknown origin, 183
Endoscopy
 for fever of unknown origin, 182
 for inflammatory bowel disease, 220–221
Enterography, CT, for inflammatory bowel disease, 221–222

F

FDG- PET and FDG-PET/CT, for infections and inflammation
 arthroplasty-associated, **139–150**, 168–169, 238–239
 fever of unknown origin, **181–189**, 213–214
 in diabetic foot, **151–160**
 inflammatory bowel disease, **219–225**
 malignancy-associated, 185, **211–218**
 osteomyelitis. *See* Osteomyelitis.
 sarcoidosis, 184, **191–210**
 therapy response, **233–243**
 vasculitis. *See* Vasculitis.
Fever of unknown origin, **181–189**
 classification of, 181–182
 imaging modalities for, 182
 in malignancy, 213–214
 PET and PET/CT for, 182–187, 213–214

PET Clin 7 (2012) 245–247
doi:10.1016/S1556-8598(12)00046-6
1556-8598/12/$ – see front matter © 2012 Elsevier Inc. All rights reserved

Moving?

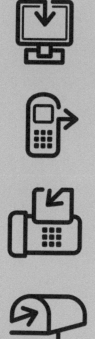

Make sure your subscription moves with you!

To notify us of your new address, find your **Clinics Account Number** (located on your mailing label above your name), and contact customer service at:

Email: journalscustomerservice-usa@elsevier.com

800-654-2452 (subscribers in the U.S. & Canada)
314-447-8871 (subscribers outside of the U.S. & Canada)

Fax number: 314-447-8029

Elsevier Health Sciences Division
Subscription Customer Service
3251 Riverport Lane
Maryland Heights, MO 63043

*To ensure uninterrupted delivery of your subscription, please notify us at least 4 weeks in advance of move.

Printed and bound by CPI Group (UK) Ltd, Croydon, CR0 4YY

03/10/2024

01040351-0007